The

ANTI-INFLAMMATORY DIET COOKBOOK

500 Healthy Recipes to Reduce Inflammation and Heal the Immune System

Michelle Moreno

ISBN 9798695420159

Table of contents

What is the Anti-Inflammatory Diet?

The anti-inflammatory diet is the best choice for your health if you have conditions that cause inflammation. Such conditions are asthma, chronic peptic ulcer, tuberculosis, rheumatoid arthritis, periodontitis, Crohn's disease, sinusitis, active hepatitis, etc. Along with medical treatment, proper nutrition is very important. An anti-inflammatory diet can help to reduce the pain from inflammation for a few notches. Such a diet isn't a panacea but a significant help in any treatment.

Inflammation is a natural response of your body to infections, injuries, and illnesses. The classic symptoms of inflammation are redness, pain, heat, and swelling. Nevertheless, some diseases don't occur any symptoms. Such illnesses are diabetes, heart disease, cancer, etc. That's why we should care about our health permanently and an anti-inflammatory diet is one of the ways for it.

The anti-inflammatory diet helps to enrich the organism with antioxidants. They help to reduce the level of free radicals in our bodies. The most common question that people ask is what to eat while the anti-inflammatory diet. As usual, the diet is varied and includes many fruits, vegetables, whole grains, plant-based proteins (legumes and nuts), fat types of fish, a lot of spices, condiments, and dressings. The only condition that should be followed is that all food should be organic. The most popular vegetables and fruits while the anti-inflammatory diet is leafy greens, cherries, raspberries, blackberries, tomatoes, cucumbers, etc. If we talk about whole grains, these are oatmeal, brown rice, and all grains that are high in fiber. Herbs and spices are natural antioxidants that will boost your health and flavor your meal. During the diet, you should avoid highly processed food (sugary drinks, chocolate, ice cream, French fries, burgers, sausages, deli meats), and overly greasy food. One more factor that will help you while anti-inflammatory treatment is the correct amount of water consumed per day. It is easy to count. There are a lot of apps that will help you to do it correctly. By drinking enough water, we help the body to cleanse faster.

As you noticed, the anti-inflammatory diet is simple to follow and is not strict much. You are free to adjust the diet by your preferences. Nevertheless, there are some cons that you should know. The anti-inflammatory diet can be costly as you need to eat preferably organic food. Likewise, the diet contains a lot of allergens such as nuts, seeds, and soy.

However, eating the right adjusted food will help to eliminate the cons of the diet. It is highly recommended to consult the doctor and make the complete medical examination before starting the diet. By doing this, you can avoid exacerbations and unwanted effects of diet.

This is the most important information that you should know before starting a diet. Any diet is not a magic remedy for all diseases; it is a support for the body during a difficult time of treatment. Start your new healthy life from one small step and you will see the huge results within half a year. You can be sure that your body will be thankful to you by giving you a fresh look and energy for new achievements.

What to Eat and Avoid on the Anti-Inflammatory Diet

Meat, Poultry and Fish

The best choice for an anti-inflammatory diet is fish and seafood. This type of food is rich in omega-3 fatty acids. It almost doesn't occur allergy reactions. Meat can be eating in moderation. Nevertheless, it is recommended to eat grass-fed meat.

What to eat	Enjoy occasionally	What to avoid
- Turkey	- Beef	- Lamb
- Tuna		- Lard
- Sole		- Chicken
- Shrimps		- Pork
- Halibut		- Bacon
- Trout		- Breaded fish
- Salmon		
- Flounder		
- Mackerel		
- Oysters		
- Sardines		
- catfish		
- clams		
- cod		
- crab		
- herring		
- lobster		
- Mahi Mahi		

Dairy

Dairy products can be both useful and harmful to your health. Full-fat dairy products can cause acne and increase inflammatory conditions. Scientifically proved that consumption of dairy products should be reduced to a minimum after 33 years old.

What to eat	Enjoy occasionally	What to avoid
- Non-fat milk	- Rice milk	- Whole cream
- Low-fat milk	- Skim milk	- Sour cream
- Coconut milk	- Tofu cheese	- Cream
- Greek-style Yogurt	- Parmesan	- Hard cheese
- Fat-free plain traditional yogurt		- Milk butter
- Cashew butter		- Margarine
- Sunflower seeds butter		- Cottage cheese

Oils and Fats

It is recommended to consume vegetable oils and fats during the anti-inflammatory diet. Bear in mind that some natural oils can cause allergy.

What to eat	Enjoy occasionally	What to avoid
- Sunflower oil (cold-pressed)	- Walnut oil	- Coconut oil
- Grapeseed oil		- Palm oil
- Olive oil (extra virgin)		
- Flax seeds oil		

Nuts and Seeds

Nuts and seeds are useful for heart health, besides this, they are rich in fiber and have nutrition features. Stop eating nuts and seeds if you have personal intolerance of them.

What to eat	Enjoy occasionally	What to avoid
- Almonds - Chia seeds - Flaxseeds - Pumpkin seeds - Pistachios - Almonds	- Hazelnuts	- Cashews - Chocolate-covered nuts - Nut butter (sweetened/ unsweetened) - Macadamia nuts - Nut butter (unsweetened) - Peanuts - Pecans - Walnuts

Vegetables

The main source of vitamins during the anti-inflammatory diet is vegetables. However, not all vegetables can bring benefits to your body. Avoid starchy vegetables and vegetables that can cause allergic reactions.

What to eat	Enjoy occasionally	What to avoid
- Sweet potatoes - Yams - Beet - Radish - Watermelon - Green beans - Organic baked corn chips - Sweet pepper - Shiitake mushrooms	- Tomatoes - Tomatillos	- Potato - Corn - Potato chips - Bell peppers - Champignon

Fruits and Berries

Fruits are rich in vitamins. Nevertheless, avoid eating large amounts of sugary fruits. Replace them with sweet and sour or sour fruits/berries.

What to eat	Enjoy occasionally	What to avoid
- Tart cherries - Strawberries - Blueberries - Apples - Pears - Apricots - Avocado - Dried fruits	- Eat all fruits that were not listed here, in moderation	- Orange - Mango - Pineapple - Papaya - Bananas

Eggs

Eggs contain essential nutrients, proteins, lutein, zeaxanthin that hold back the inflammation. Nevertheless, frequent consumption of eggs can cause allergic reactions.

Condiments

Condiments play a significant role in the meal taste. They are can make it tender, spicy, or salty. During an anti-inflammatory diet, you can use almost all spices and herbs. They have strong anti-inflammatory features.

What to eat	What to avoid
- Low-fat mayonnaise	- Mayonnaise
- Ground pink peppercorns	- Paprika
- Turmeric tahini dressing	- Tartar sauce
- Alfredo sauce	- Teriyaki
- Hot red pepper sauce	- Tomato sauce
- Turmeric tahini dressing	- Bordelaise sauce
- Chimichurri sauce	- Brown sauce
- Curry powder	- Chili sauce
- Tapatio sauce (handmade)	- Dijon sauce
- Apple cider vinegar	- Buffalo sauce
- Pomegranate sauce	- Hollandaise sauce
	- Marinara sauce
	- Tomato sauce
	- Worcestershire sauce
	- Sweet and sour sauce
	- Soy sauce
	- Pickle relish
	- Barbecue sauce
	- Mustard

Grain Products

Whole-grains are rich in fiber and can fight with inflammation and protect our body from infects. Avoid eating "bad" grains.

What to eat	What to avoid
- Brown rice	- White rice
- Wild rice	- Sugar cereals
- Oatmeal	- White bread
- Whole-grain bread	- Crackers
- Multigrain bread	- Snacks
- Whole-grain pasta	- Rye bread
- Oat flour	- Wheat noodles
- Buckwheat flour	- White bread crumbs
- Whole wheat flour	- Cornflour
- Rice noodles	- Wheat tortillas
- Corn tortillas	- Bagel
- Whole-grain toasts	

Beans and Legumes

Consumption of beans and legumes is very important during the anti-inflammatory diet. They are rich in fiber and contain the high amount of proteins. Besides this, this type of food includes a lot of antioxidants. It is necessary to eat at least 2 servings of beans or legumes per week.

Note that beans and legumes can cause inflammation only if they are cooked in the wrong way. It is recommended to soak beans before cooking.

Beverages

Drinking water should be a rule for you during the anti-inflammatory diet. Nevertheless, not all drinks can be useful to you. Avoid consuming sparkling drinks and beverages that contain artificial sugars.

What to eat	Enjoy occasionally	What to avoid
- Seltzer - Filtered water - Mineral water - Lemon water - Herbal tea - Green tea - Mate tea	- Fresh juice	- Coffee - Sodas - Wine - Sparkling mineral water - Carbonated drinks - Sweet sparkling beverages

Sweets

Fruits are the best sweets during the anti-inflammatory diet. They are rich in vitamins and contain only natural sweeteners.

Nevertheless, you can find a lot of sugar-free meals which are not inferior in taste to the most famous desserts.

What to eat	Enjoy occasionally	What to avoid
- Honey - Raw cocoa powder - Fruits (allowed for anti-inflammatory diet)	- Stevia - Xylitol - Brown rice syrup - Black chocolate	- Artificial sweeteners - Buns - Candy - Cakes - Chocolate - Cookies - Custard - Ice cream - Pastries - Pies - Pudding - Sugar - Tarts - Corn syrup - Milk chocolate

Others

Fast food and processed food are forbidden during the anti-inflammatory diet. Such food damages our gut system and reduces the protective qualities of our body and, as a result, destroy the immune system.

What to avoid
- Fried foods - Processed foods

Top 10 Anti-Inflammatory Diet Tips

1. Avoid white food.
Avoiding white food such as sugar, salt, etc. can help to maintain and control the normal level of blood sugar. Try to add more lean proteins and high fiber food in your daily diet. It can be lean types of meat, brown rice, and whole grains.

2. An apple a day keeps the doctors away.
Add vegetables, fruits, nuts, and spices in your daily meal plan. Garlic, ginger, cinnamon, and lemon will help to boost your immune system and reduce inflammation.

3. Do sport daily.
Regular sports activities can help to prevent inflammation. Make 5-10-minute sport exercises daily to feel healthier.

4. Balance your mind.
Everyday stress leads to the most chronic diseases. Practicing yoga, meditation or biofeedback are excellent ways to balance your mind and manage stress.

5. Choose the right proteins.
Lean red meat can be served as a source of proteins but still, it is high in cholesterol and salt. Instead of it, choose fish such as halibut, salmon, tuna, cod, or seabass. They are rich in omega-3 fatty acids.

6. Drink antioxidant beverages.
Herbs are a great source of antioxidants and promote faster treatment. Basil, thyme, oregano, chili pepper, and curcumin have high anti-inflammatory features and serve as natural painkillers:

7. Control the sleeping time.
Eight-nine hours for sleeping should be a rule for you. Less sleep and oversleep are the main triggers for heart disease and 2-type diabetes.

8. Cross out alcohol from your diet.
Refusing from alcohol helps to make the body calm and reduce the risk of inflammation.

9. Choose green tea instead of coffee and tea.
Green tea can fight with free radical damage. Regular drinking of green tea lowers the risk of cancer and Alzheimer's disease.

10. Consume the probiotic every day.
Urban lifestyle and junk food damage our gut. Its health is very important. Try to eat food that is rich in probiotics every day. Doing this, you will improve the gut's microbe barrier. Such food is sauerkraut, yogurt, milk, kombucha, miso, kimchi, and fermented vegetables/fruits.

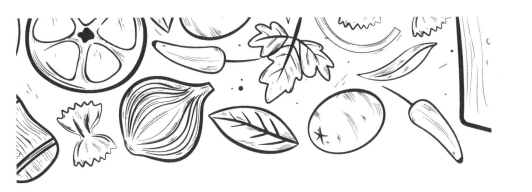

Breakfast

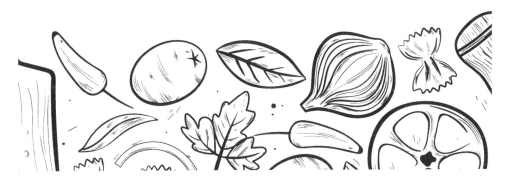

Garlic Pork

Prep time: 10 minutes | **Servings:** 4
Cook time: 1 hour

- 1-pound pork tenderloin
- 2 tablespoons avocado oil
- 1 tablespoon minced garlic
- ¼ cup of water
- ½ teaspoon cayenne pepper

1. Pour water in the baking pan.
2. Then rub the pork tenderloin with avocado oil, minced garlic, and cayenne pepper.
3. Put the meat in the pan with water and bake at 375F for 1 hour.

per serving: 175 calories, 29.9g protein, 1.2g carbohydrates, 4.9g fat, 0.4g fiber, 83mg cholesterol, 66mg sodium, 513mg potassium.

Yam Salad

Prep time: 10 minutes | **Servings:** 2
Cook time: 0 minutes

- 1 tablespoon olive oil
- 1 cup spinach, chopped
- 1 tomato, chopped
- 8 oz yams, peeled, chopped, boiled

1. Mix yams with tomato and spinach.
2. Sprinkle the salad with olive oil and gently shake.

per serving: 201 calories, 2.4g protein, 32.9g carbohydrates, 7.3g fat, 5.1g fiber, 0mg cholesterol, 22mg sodium, 917mg potassium.

Vanilla Pears

Prep time: 10 minutes | **Servings:** 4
Cook time: 15 minutes

- 2 cups of rice milk
- 4 pears, chopped
- 1 teaspoon vanilla extract

1. Bring the rice milk to boil.
2. Add vanilla extract and chopped pears.
3. Simmer the meal for 5 minutes on medium heat.

per serving: 184 calories, 1g protein, 44.4g carbohydrates, 1.3g fat, 6.5g fiber, 0mg cholesterol, 45mg sodium, 278mg potassium.

Yam Cakes

Prep time: 10 minutes | **Servings:** 6
Cook time: 10 minutes

- 1 cup almond flour
- 1 oz brown rice, cooked
- 1 tablespoon flax meal
- 1 teaspoon baking soda
- 2 eggs, beaten
- 1 small yellow onion, chopped
- 1 teaspoon cayenne pepper
- 1 tablespoon olive oil
- 7 oz yams, peeled, grated

1. Mix yams with almond flour, brown rice, flax meal, baking soda, eggs, onion, and cayenne pepper.
2. Make the medium-size cakes.
3. Line the baking tray with baking paper.
4. Put the yam cakes inside and sprinkle them with olive oil.
5. Bake the yam cakes at 400F for 10 minutes.

per serving: 219 calories, 7.1g protein, 18.4g carbohydrates, 13.3g fat, 4.1g fiber, 55mg cholesterol, 241mg sodium, 286mg potassium.

Turmeric Cream

Prep time: 10 minutes | **Servings:** 2
Cook time: 30 minutes

- 1 cup coconut cream
- 4 eggs, beaten
- 1 tablespoon ground turmeric
- 1 teaspoon vanilla extract

1. Mix coconut cream with eggs and ground turmeric.
2. Add vanilla extract. Gently mix the mixture.
3. Pour it in the baking ramekins and transfer in the preheated to 365F oven.
4. Cook the cream for 30 minutes.

per serving: 420 calories, 14.1g protein, 9.8g carbohydrates, 37.7g fat, 3.4g fiber, 327mg cholesterol, 143mg sodium, 522mg potassium.

Fruit Bowl

Prep time: 10 minutes | **Servings:** 2
Cook time: 0 minutes

- 2 oranges, peeled, chopped
- 1 banana, chopped
- 2 kiwis, peeled, chopped
- 1 teaspoon poppy
- seeds
- 1 tablespoon coconut cream
- 1 teaspoon coconut shred

1. Mix oranges with a banana in a salad bowl.
2. Add kiwis, poppy seeds, and coconut shred. Gently shake the mixture.
3. Top the meal with coconut cream.

per serving: 218 calories,3.7g protein, 47.3g carbohydrates, 4.1g fat, 8.7g fiber, 0mg cholesterol, 5mg sodium, 811mg potassium.

Golden Milk

Prep time: 10 minutes | **Servings:** 2
Cook time: 15 minutes

- 2 cups of coconut milk
- 2 tablespoons
- ground turmeric
- ½ teaspoon ground cinnamon

1. Bring the coconut milk to boil.
2. Then add ground cinnamon and turmeric. Whisk the liquid until it is smooth.
3. Simmer it for 1 minute and pour in the serving glasses.

per serving: 578 calories,6.1g protein, 18.2g carbohydrates, 57.9g fat, 7g fiber, 0mg cholesterol, 39mg sodium, 805mg potassium.

Strawberry Salad

Prep time: 5 minutes | **Servings:** 1
Cook time: 0 minutes

- 2 oz nuts, chopped
- 1 cup strawberries, sliced
- 2 tablespoons
- coconut milk
- 1 teaspoon coconut shred

1. Mix nuts with strawberries and coconut shred.
2. Top the salad with coconut milk.

per serving: 469 calories,11.5g protein,27.8g carbohydrates, 38.4g fat, 9g fiber, 0mg cholesterol, 386mg sodium, 638mg potassium.

Vanilla Pudding

Prep time: 10 minutes | **Servings:** 3
Cook time: 0 minutes

- 2 cups plain yogurt
- 4 tablespoons chia seeds, dried
- ½ cup strawberries, sliced
- 1 teaspoon vanilla extract

1. Mix plain yogurt with vanilla extract, and chia seeds and leave for 15 minutes.
2. Then transfer the pudding in the serving glasses and top with strawberries.

per serving: 216 calories,12.6g protein, 21.3g carbohydrates, 7.9g fat, 7g fiber, 10mg cholesterol, 118mg sodium, 496mg potassium.

Ginger Pork Chops

Prep time: 10 minutes | **Servings:** 4
Cook time: 40 minutes

- 4 pork chops
- 1 teaspoon minced ginger
- ½ teaspoon ground ginger
- 1 tablespoon olive oil
- 1 teaspoon lemon juice
- ¼ cup of water

1. Rub the pork chops with minced ginger, ground ginger, olive oil, and lemon juice.
2. Then put the pork chops in casserole mold.
3. Add water and cover the mold with foil.
4. Bake the pork chops at 375F for 40 minutes.

per serving: 288 calories,18g protein, 0.4g carbohydrates, 23.4g fat, 0.1g fiber, 69mg cholesterol, 57mg sodium, 283mg potassium.

Pumpkin Pie Spices Quinoa

Prep time: 10 minutes | **Servings:** 4
Cook time: 0 minutes

- 2 cups quinoa, cooked
- 1 tablespoon pumpkin pie
- spices
- 1 tablespoon raw honey

1. Mix quinoa with pumpkin pie spices.
2. Top the meal with raw honey.

per serving: 334 calories,12.1g protein, 59.9g carbohydrates, 5.3g fat, 6.2g fiber, 0mg cholesterol, 5mg sodium, 491mg potassium.

Cashew Porridge

Prep time: 10 minutes | **Servings:** 2
Cook time: 0 minutes

- 1 cup cashew milk, warm
- 1 cup apricots, chopped
- ½ cup quinoa, cooked
- ¼ cup pistachios, chopped
- 2 teaspoons raw honey

1. Mix quinoa with cashew milk.
2. Transfer the mixture in the serving bowls.
3. Top the quinoa with apricots, pistachios, and raw honey.

per serving: 285 calories,8.5g protein, 48g carbohydrates, 7.8g fat, 5.2g fiber, 0mg cholesterol, 129mg sodium, 536mg potassium.

Winter Salad

Prep time: 10 minutes | **Servings:** 6
Cook time: 0 minutes

- 1 cup carrot, grated
- 1 oz raisins, chopped
- 3 apples, grated
- 1 tablespoon raw honey
- 3 oz celery root, grated
- 1 tablespoon olive oil

1. In the mixing bowl, mix grated carrot with raisins, apples, and celery root.
2. Then add olive oil and honey.
3. Carefully mix the salad with the help of the spoon.

per serving: 116 calories,0.8g protein, 25.1g carbohydrates, 2.6g fat, 3.6g fiber, 0mg cholesterol, 28mg sodium, 258mg potassium.

Parsley Frittata

Prep time: 10 minutes | **Servings:** 4
Cook time: 20 minutes

- ¼ cup plain yogurt
- 6 eggs, beaten
- ½ cup parsley, chopped
- 1 teaspoon olive oil
- ½ teaspoon cayenne pepper

1. Mix plain yogurt with eggs, parsley, and cayenne pepper.
2. Then pour the olive oil in the skillet and preheat it well.

3. Pour the egg mixture in the skillet, flatten it gently and close the lid.
4. Cook the frittata over the medium heat for 20 minutes.

per serving: 119 calories,9.4g protein, 2.2g carbohydrates, 8g fat, 0.3g fiber, 246mg cholesterol, 107mg sodium, 170mg potassium.

Raisins Muesli

Prep time: 10 minutes | **Servings:** 4
Cook time: 0 minutes

- 1 cup apricots, chopped
- 1 cup rolled oats
- 3 oz raisins
- 3 tablespoons chia seeds
- 2 cups of coconut milk
- ½ cup goji berries
- 4 teaspoons raw honey
- ½ teaspoon ground cinnamon

1. Mix raisins with rolled oats.
2. Add chia seeds, goji berries, and ground cinnamon. Mix the mixture.
3. Then add apricots, coconut milk, and raw honey.
4. Gently stir the muesli.

per serving: 589 calories,9.1g protein, 69.2g carbohydrates, 34.7g fat, 12.2g fiber, 0mg cholesterol, 24mg sodium, 697mg potassium.

Pepper Eggs

Prep time: 10 minutes | **Servings:** 2
Cook time: 10 minutes

- 1 cup bell pepper, chopped
- 4 eggs, beaten
- 1 teaspoon olive oil
- ½ teaspoon cayenne pepper

1. Preheat the olive oil in the skillet.
2. Then add peppers and roast them for 2-3 minutes.
3. Add eggs and cayenne pepper.
4. Gently stir the egg mixture and cook it for 7 minutes on medium heat.

per serving: 166 calories,11.7g protein, 5.4g carbohydrates, 11.3g fat, 0.9g fiber, 327mg cholesterol, 125mg sodium, 239mg potassium.

Pistachios Salad

Prep time: 10 minutes | **Servings:** 2
Cook time: 0 minutes

- ½ cup tomatoes, chopped
- 1 cucumber, chopped
- 1 sweet pepper, chopped
- ½ cup fresh cilantro, chopped
- 2 oz pistachios, chopped
- 1 tablespoon lemon juice
- 1 tablespoon olive oil

1. Put all ingredients in the salad bowl.
2. Gently shake the salad.

per serving: 264 calories,7.8g protein, 19.6g carbohydrates, 20.7g fat, 5.1g fiber, 0mg cholesterol, 161mg sodium, 763mg potassium.

Blueberry Bowl

Prep time: 10 minutes | **Servings:** 2
Cook time: 0 minutes

- 1 avocado, peeled, pitted, chopped
- 1 cup blueberries
- ½ cup of coconut milk
- 1 tablespoon coconut shred

1. Mix avocado with blueberries.
2. Then add coconut milk and coconut shred.
3. Gently stir the meal.

per serving: 410 calories,3.8g protein, 23.5g carbohydrates, 36.7g fat, 10.3g fiber, 0mg cholesterol, 17mg sodium, 701mg potassium.

Portuguese Salad

Prep time: 10 minutes | **Servings:** 4
Cook time: 0 minutes

- 3 cups tomatoes, sliced
- 2 red onions, peeled, sliced
- 2 tablespoons olive oil
- ½ teaspoon cayenne pepper

1. Mix tomatoes with red onions, and cayenne pepper.
2. Then top the salad with olive oil and stir it before serving.

per serving: 107 calories,1.8g protein, 10.5g carbohydrates, 7.4g fat, 2.9g fiber, 0mg cholesterol, 9mg sodium, 405mg potassium.

Spinach Frittata

Prep time: 10 minutes | **Servings:** 4
Cook time: 30 minutes

- 2 cups spinach, chopped
- 6 eggs, beaten
- 1 tablespoon cashew butter
- 1 teaspoon chili powder
- ¼ cup coconut cream

1. Mix all ingredients except cashew butter in the mixing bowl.
2. Then grease the baking pan with cashew butter and pour the egg mixture inside.
3. Bake the frittata at 350F for 30 minutes.

per serving: 158 calories,9.9g protein, 29g carbohydrates, 3.3g fat, 12.3g fiber, 246mg cholesterol, 144mg sodium, 246mg potassium.

Cabbage Salad

Prep time: 15 minutes | **Servings:** 4
Cook time: 0 minutes

- 2 cucumbers, chopped
- 4 cups white cabbage, shredded
- 3 tablespoons olive oil
- 2 tablespoons lemon juice
- 2 tablespoons fresh dill, chopped

1. Mix all ingredients in the salad bowl and leave for 10 minutes to marinate.

per serving: 136 calories,2.3g protein, 10.6g carbohydrates, 10.9g fat, 2.7g fiber, 0mg cholesterol, 20mg sodium, 401mg potassium.

Granola Bars

Prep time: 20 minutes | **Servings:** 4
Cook time: 0 minutes

- 7 oz pistachios, chopped
- 1 cup dates, pitted
- ½ cup raisins,
- chopped
- 2 tablespoons chia seeds

1. Mix all ingredients in the bowl.
2. When the mixture is homogenous, transfer it in the baking paper and flatten it in the shape of a square.
3. Cut the granola into bars.

per serving: 479 calories,12.7g protein, 64g carbohydrates, 25.6g fat, 11.6g fiber, 0mg cholesterol, 269mg sodium, 969mg potassium.

Tomato Eggs

Prep time: 10 minutes | **Servings:** 6
Cook time: 15 minutes

- 12 eggs, beaten
- 2 cups tomatoes, chopped
- 2 tablespoons olive oil
- 1 teaspoon dried rosemary
- ½ teaspoon chili powder

1. Preheat the olive oil in the skillet.
2. Add tomatoes, dried rosemary, and chili powder.
3. Roast tomatoes for 10 minutes. Stir them from time to time.
4. After this, add eggs, gently stir the meal and cook it for 5 minutes more with the closed lid.

per serving: 178 calories,11.6g protein, 29g carbohydrates, 3.3g fat, 13.6g fiber, 327mg cholesterol, 128mg sodium, 266mg potassium.

Italian Style Salad

Prep time: 10 minutes | **Servings:** 4
Cook time: 0 minutes

- 1 tablespoon Italian seasonings
- 2 tablespoons olive oil
- 2 oz Parmesan, grated
- 2 oz olives, chopped
- 1 cup tomatoes, chopped
- 1 cup cucumbers, chopped

1. Mix olives with tomatoes and cucumbers.
2. Then sprinkle the salad with Italian seasonings and olive oil.
3. Shake the salad.
4. Top it with parmesan.

per serving: 145 calories,5.3g protein, 4.5g carbohydrates, 12.7g fat, 1.1g fiber, 13mg cholesterol, 259mg sodium, 148mg potassium.

Zucchini Eggs

Prep time: 10 minutes | **Servings:** 2
Cook time: 15 minutes

- 1 zucchini, spiralized
- 1 tablespoon olive oil
- 1 teaspoon dried rosemary
- ¼ cup plain yogurt
- 2 eggs, beaten

1. Preheat the olive oil in the skillet.
2. Add eggs and top them with dried rosemary.
3. Cook the eggs for 3 minutes on low heat.
4. After this, add zucchini and plain yogurt.
5. Mix the mixture gently, close the lid, and cook it on low heat for 12 minutes.

per serving: 162 calories,8.5g protein, 6.2g carbohydrates, 12g fat, 1.3g fiber, 166mg cholesterol, 93mg sodium, 393mg potassium.

Kale Salad

Prep time: 10 minutes | **Servings:** 4
Cook time: 0 minutes

- 3 cups kale, chopped
- 2 cucumbers, chopped
- ¼ cup fresh parsley, chopped
- 2 tablespoons lemon juice
- ½ teaspoon dried mint
- 3 oz tofu, cubed

1. Mix kale with cucumbers and parsley.
2. Then sprinkle the salad with lemon juice and dried mint.
3. Shake the salad and top it with tofu.

per serving: 66 calories,4.4g protein, 11.5g carbohydrates, 1.2g fat, 1.9g fiber, 0mg cholesterol, 31mg sodium, 531mg potassium.

Quinoa Salad

Prep time: 10 minutes | **Servings:** 2
Cook time: 0 minutes

- 2 cups quinoa, cooked
- 1 cup tomatoes, chopped
- 1 cup fresh parsley, chopped
- 1 tablespoon olive oil
- 1 teaspoon lemon juice
- 2 garlic cloves, diced

1. In the salad bowl, mix quinoa with tomatoes, parsley, and garlic cloves.
2. Then add olive oil and lemon juice.
3. Stir the salad.

per serving: 718 calories,25.9g protein, 115.5g carbohydrates, 17.8g fat, 14g fiber, 0mg cholesterol, 31mg sodium, 1352mg potassium.

Shredded Carrot Bowl

Prep time: 10 minutes | **Servings:** 4
Cook time: 0 minutes

- 3 cups carrot, shredded
- 3 oz raisins, chopped
- 3 tablespoons lemon juice
- 2 tablespoons olive oil
- 1 tablespoons dried cilantro
- 1 tablespoon raw honey

1. Put all ingredients in the salad bowl and carefully mix.
2. Let the meal rest for at least 5 minutes before serving.

per serving: 176 calories,1.5g protein, 29.9g carbohydrates, 7.2g fat, 2.9g fiber, 0mg cholesterol, 62mg sodium, 441mg potassium.

Sprouts Salad

Prep time: 10 minutes | **Servings:** 4
Cook time: 0 minutes

- 1 red onion, sliced
- 2 cups bean sprouts
- 1 cup fresh cilantro, chopped
- 1 tablespoon
- lemon juice
- 1 teaspoon dried rosemary
- 1 tablespoon olive oil

1. Put all ingredients in the salad bowl.
2. Shake the salad well.

per serving: 71 calories,4.3g protein, 6.8g carbohydrates, 4.1g fat, 0.9g fiber, 0mg cholesterol, 9mg sodium, 241mg potassium.

Corn Bowl

Prep time: 10 minutes | **Servings:** 4
Cook time: 0 minutes

- 10 oz corn kernels, cooked
- 1 cup tomatoes, chopped
- 1 tablespoon fresh
- dill, chopped
- 1 tablespoon plain yogurt
- ½ cup radish, chopped

1. Mix tomatoes with fresh dill, plain yogurt, and radish.
2. Then add corn kernels, gently stir the meal.

per serving: 345 calories,13.4g protein, 75.5g carbohydrates, 4.7g fat, 11.4g fiber, 0mg cholesterol, 70mg sodium, 1215mg potassium.

Lemon Tomatoes

Prep time: 10 minutes | **Servings:** 6
Cook time: 0 minutes

- 4 cups arugula, chopped
- 4 cups tomatoes, chopped
- 2 tablespoons olive
- oil
- 3 tablespoons lemon juice
- 1 teaspoon lemon zest, grated

1. Put tomatoes and arugula in the salad bowl.
2. Add lemon juice, olive oil, and lemon zest.
3. Stir the meal gently before serving.

per serving: 67 calories,1.5g protein, 5.4g carbohydrates, 5.1g fat, 1.7g fiber, 0mg cholesterol, 11mg sodium, 344mg potassium.

Watermelon Salad

Prep time: 10 minutes | **Servings:** 2
Cook time: 0 minutes

- 4 oz Romano cheese, grated
- 10 oz watermelon, chopped
- 2 oz raisins, chopped
- 1 tablespoon coconut cream

1. Put the watermelon in the bowl and top it with cheese and raisins.
2. Then sprinkle the salad with coconut cream.

per serving: 364 calories,19.9g protein, 35.6g carbohydrates, 17.4g fat, 1.8g fiber, 59mg cholesterol, 687mg sodium, 438mg potassium.

Lettuce Salad

Prep time: 5 minutes | **Servings:** 2
Cook time: 0 minutes

- 2 cups lettuce, chopped
- 1 cup raspberries
- 1 tablespoon chia seeds
- 1 tablespoon olive oil
- ½ teaspoon ground cinnamon

1. Mix lettuce with raspberries, olive oil, and ground cinnamon.
2. Top the salad with chia seeds.

per serving: 135 calories,2.2g protein, 12.4g carbohydrates, 9.7g fat, 7.1g fiber, 0mg cholesterol, 5mg sodium, 202mg potassium.

Avocado Salad

Prep time: 10 minutes | **Servings:** 4
Cook time: 0 minutes

- 3 tomatoes, roughly chopped
- 2 avocados, pitted and chopped
- 1 cup parsley, chopped
- 1 teaspoon cayenne pepper
- ½ teaspoon dried rosemary
- 2 tablespoons olive oil

1. In the salad bowl, mix tomatoes with avocados, parsley, and dried rosemary.
2. Then sprinkle the salad with olive oil and cayenne pepper. Gently shake the salad.

per serving: 289 calories, 3.2g protein, 13.5g carbohydrates, 27g fat, 8.5g fiber, 0mg cholesterol, 19mg sodium, 800mg potassium.

Blueberry Porridge

Prep time: 10 minutes | **Servings:** 4
Cook time: 0 minutes

- 4 tablespoons chia seeds
- 1 cup blueberries
- 3 cups coconut cream
- 4 teaspoons raw honey
- ½ teaspoon vanilla extract

1. Mix coconut cream with chis seeds and raw honey.
2. Blend the blueberries until smooth and add in the chia mixture.
3. Then add vanilla extract, stir the porridge, and transfer in the serving bowls.

per serving: 526 calories, 6.8g protein, 27g carbohydrates, 47.4g fat, 9.7g fiber, 0mg cholesterol, 30mg sodium, 563mg potassium.

Garlic Pork Chops

Prep time: 10 minutes | **Servings:** 4
Cook time: 10 minutes

- 4 pork chops
- 1 tablespoon minced garlic
- 1 tomato, crushed
- 1 tablespoon olive oil

1. Rub the pork chops with minced garlic and crushed tomato.
2. Then sprinkle the meat with olive oil.
3. Grill the pork chops at 400F for 5 minutes per side.

per serving: 292 calories, 18.3g protein, 1.3g carbohydrates, 23.4g fat, 0.2g fiber, 69mg cholesterol, 57mg sodium, 320mg potassium.

Banana Porridge

Prep time: 5 minutes | **Servings:** 6
Cook time: 5 minutes

- 8 bananas, peeled, chopped
- 4 tablespoons chia seeds
- 1 cup coconut cream
- 1 teaspoon vanilla extract

1. Preheat the coconut cream until warm.
2. Add chopped bananas and chia seeds.
3. Then add vanilla extract, gently stir the porridge, and transfer in the serving plates/bowls.

per serving: 280 calories, 4.2g protein, 42.2g carbohydrates, 13g fat, 8.2g fiber, 0mg cholesterol, 9mg sodium, 708mg potassium.

Apple Oats

Prep time: 20 minutes | **Servings:** 2
Cook time: 0 minutes

- 1 cup old-fashioned oats
- ½ cup of coconut milk
- 1 tablespoon
- maple syrup
- 2 apples, chopped
- 1 oz pistachios, chopped

1. Mix oats with coconut milk and maple syrup and leave for 15 minutes.
2. Then add apples and pistachios.
3. Stir the meal.

per serving: 506 calories, 10.1g protein, 71.6g carbohydrates, 24g fat, 12.1g fiber, 0mg cholesterol, 89mg sodium, 708mg potassium.

Beet Noodles Salad

Prep time: 5 minutes | **Servings:** 4
Cook time: 0 minutes

- 2 cups beets, baked, spiralized
- 1 cup spinach, chopped
- 2 tablespoons olive
- oil
- 1 red onion, peeled, chopped
- 1 cup tomatoes, chopped

1. Mix beets with spinach, onion, and tomatoes,
2. Shake the mixture gently and top it with olive oil.

per serving: 118 calories, 2.3g protein, 13.1g carbohydrates, 7.3g fat, 3g fiber, 0mg cholesterol, 75mg sodium, 448mg potassium.

Nutmeg Oats

Prep time: 15 minutes | **Servings:** 2
Cook time: 10 minutes

- 1 cup of coconut milk
- ½ cup old-fashioned oats
- 1 pear, chopped
- 1 teaspoon ground nutmeg
- 2 teaspoons raw honey

1. Bring the coconut milk to boil and add oats.
2. Simmer them for 5 minutes.
3. Then remove the oats from the heat and add pear, ground nutmeg, and honey.
4. Gently stir the meal.

per serving: 418 calories, 5.7g protein, 37g carbohydrates, 30.4g fat, 7g fiber, 0mg cholesterol, 20mg sodium, 476mg potassium.

Pineapple Bowl

Prep time: 5 minutes | **Servings:** 2
Cook time: 0 minutes

- 1 cup pineapple, peeled and cubed
- 1 avocado, peeled, chopped
- 1 pear, cubed
- 1 teaspoon chia seeds
- 1 tablespoon lemon juice
- ½ tablespoon avocado oil

1. In the bowl mix pineapple with avocado, pear, lemon juice, and avocado oil.
2. Shake the mixture and top with chia seeds.

per serving: 373 calories, 3.4g protein, 32.2g carbohydrates, 28.3g fat, 11.7g fiber, 0mg cholesterol, 10mg sodium, 687mg potassium.

Mango Pork

Prep time: 10 minutes | **Servings:** 4
Cook time: 40 minutes

- 4 pork chops
- 1 mango, pitted, peeled, chopped
- 1 tablespoon olive oil
- ½ teaspoon chili powder
- ¼ cup of water

1. Sprinkle the pork chops with olive oil and chili powder. Put them in the baking pan.
2. Then top the meat with water and mango.
3. Bake the meat for 40 minutes at 360F.

per serving: 337 calories, 18.7g protein, 12.8g carbohydrates, 23.8g fat, 1.5g fiber, 69mg cholesterol, 61mg sodium, 423mg potassium.

Nutmeg Pork

Prep time: 10 minutes | **Servings:** 4
Cook time: 45 minutes

- 1 tablespoon ground nutmeg
- 1 cup of water
- 1-pound pork tenderloin, chopped
- 1 teaspoon dried rosemary

1. Bring the water to boil.
2. Add ground nutmeg and dried rosemary.
3. Then add pork tenderloin and close the lid.
4. Simmer the meat on low heat for 35 minutes.

per serving: 172 calories, 29.8g protein, 1.1g carbohydrates, 4.7g fat, 0.5g fiber, 83mg cholesterol, 67mg sodium, 487mg potassium.

Pork with Shallot

Prep time: 10 minutes | **Servings:** 4
Cook time: 1 hour

- 1 pound pork meat, cubed
- 1 cup shallot, chopped
- 1 tablespoon almond butter
- 1 cup of water
- 1 teaspoon cayenne pepper

1. Pour water in the saucepan.
2. Add all remaining ingredients and close the lid.
3. Cook the meat on medium heat for 1 hour.

per serving: 433 calories, 16.1g protein, 10.1g carbohydrates, 36.7g fat, 0.5g fiber, 70mg cholesterol, 1469mg sodium, 417mg potassium.

Sweet Pork

Prep time: 10 minutes | **Servings:** 4
Cook time: 55 minutes

- 2 pounds pork stew meat, cubed
- 2 apples, chopped
- 1 tablespoon liquid honey
- 2 tablespoons almond butter
- 1 cup of water
- 1 teaspoon ground clove

1. Put all ingredients in the saucepan.
2. Stir them gently and close the lid.
3. Cook the sweet pork on medium heat for 55 minutes.

per serving: 605 calories, 68.4g protein, 21.6g carbohydrates, 26.7g fat, 3.7g fiber, 195mg cholesterol, 139mg sodium, 1039mg potassium.

Sage Pork Roast

Prep time: 10 minutes | **Servings:** 4
Cook time: 1 hour

- 2 pounds pork loin
  roast, sliced
- 1 tablespoon sage
- 1 tablespoon
  minced garlic
- 1 teaspoon
  cayenne pepper
- 2 tablespoons olive
  oil

1. Mix pork loin with sage, minced garlic, cayenne pepper, and olive oil.
2. Put the meat in the baking pan, flatten it gently, and bake at 355F for 1 hour. Stir the meat during cooking to avoid burning.

per serving: 540 calories, 65.1g protein, 1.2g carbohydrates, 29g fat, 0.4g fiber, 184mg cholesterol, 132mg sodium, 987mg potassium.

Onion Pork Roast

Prep time: 10 minutes | **Servings:** 4
Cook time: 1 hour

- 2 pounds pork
  roast, sliced
- 2 onions, peeled,
  sliced
- 2 tablespoons olive
- oil
- 1 teaspoon ground
  ginger
- ¼ cup of water

1. Preheat the olive oil in the saucepan.
2. Add pork roast and cook it for 3 minutes per side.
3. Then sprinkle the meat with ground ginger, sliced onion, and water.
4. Close the lid and cook the meal for 54 minutes on low heat.

per serving: 553 calories, 65.3g protein, 5.5g carbohydrates, 28.5g fat, 1.2g fiber, 195mg cholesterol, 130mg sodium, 998mg potassium.

Lemon Pork Chops

Prep time: 10 minutes | **Servings:** 4
Cook time: 40 minutes

- 4 pork chops
- 1 lemon, sliced
- 1 tablespoon olive
- oil
- ½ teaspoon
  ground clove

1. Brush the pork chops with olive oil from each side.
2. Then put the meat in the casserole mold and sprinkle with ground clove.
3. Top the meat with lemon and bake at 355F for 40 minutes.

per serving: 287 calories, 18g protein, 0.2g carbohydrates, 23.4g fat, 0.1g fiber, 69mg cholesterol, 57mg sodium, 280mg potassium.

Rosemary Pork Cubes

Prep time: 10 minutes | **Servings:** 4
Cook time: 40 minutes

- 2 pounds pork
  stew meat, cubed
- 1 tablespoon dried
  rosemary
- 1 cup tomatoes,
  chopped
- 4 garlic cloves,
  chopped
- 2 cups of water
- 1 tablespoon olive
  oil

1. In the mixing bowl, mix pork stew meat with dried rosemary, garlic, and olive oil.
2. Then put the mixture in the saucepan, add tomatoes and water.
3. Close the lid and cook the meal on low heat for 40 minutes.

per serving: 526 calories, 67g protein, 3.3g carbohydrates, 25.7g fat, 1g fiber, 195mg cholesterol, 140mg sodium, 978mg potassium.

Lemongrass Pork

Prep time: 10 minutes | **Servings:** 4
Cook time: 30 minutes

- 1-pound pork loin,
  roughly chopped
- 1 tablespoon
  lemongrass,
  chopped
- 1 cup coconut
- cream
- 1 teaspoon dried
  rosemary
- 1 teaspoon ground
  cinnamon

1. In the shallow bowl, mix lemongrass with dried rosemary and ground cinnamon.
2. Mix the spices with the meat and put it in the casserole mold.
3. Add coconut cream and cook the meat at 375F for 30 minutes.

per serving: 416 calories, 32.4g protein, 4.3g carbohydrates, 30.2g fat, 1.8g fiber, 91mg cholesterol, 80mg sodium, 652mg potassium.

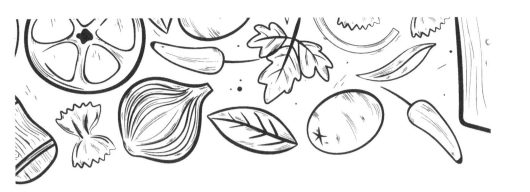

Side Dishes

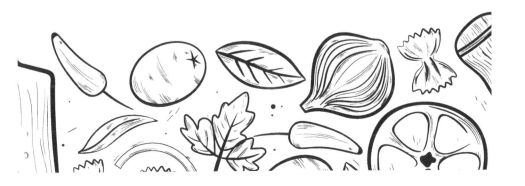

Lemon Carrots

Prep time: 10 minutes | **Servings:** 4
Cook time: 25 minutes

- 1 lemon
- 1-pound carrot, peeled, chopped
- 1 teaspoon ground
- cinnamon
- 1 tablespoon olive oil

1. Mix the carrots with ground cinnamon and olive oil.
2. Put the carrot in the baking tray.
3. Then squeeze the lemon juice over the carrots
4. Bake the carrots at 385F for 25 minutes.

per serving: 82 calories, 1.1g protein, 13g carbohydrates, 3.6g fat, 3.5g fiber, 0mg cholesterol, 78mg sodium, 385mg potassium.

Parmesan Endive

Prep time: 5 minutes | **Servings:** 4
Cook time: 15 minutes

- 1-pound endives, trimmed
- 3 oz Parmesan, grated
- 1 tablespoon olive oil
- ½ teaspoon cayenne pepper

1. Sprinkle the endives with olive oil and cayenne pepper and put in the tray.
2. Bake the endives for 10 minutes at 365F.
3. Then top the endives with Parmesan and cook for 5 minutes more.

per serving: 118 calories, 8.3g protein, 4.7g carbohydrates, 8.3g fat, 3.6g fiber, 15mg cholesterol, 222mg sodium, 361mg potassium.

Rosemary Carrots

Prep time: 10 minutes | **Servings:** 4
Cook time: 40 minutes

- 2 tablespoons olive oil
- 1-pound carrot, peeled, roughly
- chopped
- 1 tablespoon dried rosemary

1. Mix the carrots with olive oil and dried rosemary.
2. Put the vegetables in the lined with the baking paper tray and bake at 375F for 40 minutes.

per serving: 109 calories, 1g protein, 11.7g carbohydrates, 7.1g fat, 3.1g fiber, 0mg cholesterol, 79mg sodium, 370mg potassium.

Zucchini Slices

Prep time: 5 minutes | **Servings:** 4
Cook time: 20 minutes

- 4 large zucchinis, sliced
- 2 tablespoons olive oil
- ½ teaspoon
- ground black pepper
- 3 oz Parmesan, grated

1. Line the baking tray with baking paper.
2. Then put the zucchini slices in the baking tray in one layer. Sprinkle the vegetables with olive oil and ground black pepper.
3. Top the zucchinis with Parmesan and bake at 360F for 20 minutes.

per serving: 181 calories, 10.8g protein, 11.8g carbohydrates, 12.1g fat, 3.6g fiber, 15mg cholesterol, 230mg sodium, 850mg potassium.

Baked Broccoli

Prep time: 10 minutes | **Servings:** 4
Cook time: 30 minutes

- 2-pounds broccoli, roughly chopped
- 2 tablespoons olive
- oil
- 1 tablespoon cayenne pepper

1. Line the baking tray with baking paper.
2. Put the broccoli in the tray and sprinkle with olive oil and cayenne pepper.
3. Bake the broccoli for 30 minutes at 355F.

per serving: 141 calories, 6.5g protein, 15.8g carbohydrates, 8g fat, 6.3g fiber, 0mg cholesterol, 75mg sodium, 745mg potassium.

Sauteed Kale

Prep time: 10 minutes | **Servings:** 4
Cook time: 20 minutes

- 4 cups kale, chopped
- 1 cup coconut cream
- 2 oz walnuts, chopped
- 1 teaspoon dried sage

1. Mix kale with coconut cream in the saucepan.
2. Add walnuts and dried sage.
3. Close the lid and cook the meal on medium heat for 20 minutes.

per serving: 259 calories, 6.8g protein, 11.8g carbohydrates, 22.7g fat, 3.4g fiber, 0mg cholesterol, 38mg sodium, 563mg potassium.

Turmeric Mushrooms

Prep time: 10 minutes | **Servings:** 4
Cook time: 20 minutes

- 1 pound mushrooms, sliced
- 1 tablespoon ground turmeric
- ½ cup cilantro, chopped
- 1 tablespoon olive oil
- 3 garlic cloves, diced

1. Mix mushrooms with ground turmeric, cilantro, and garlic.
2. Put the mixture in the saucepan, add olive oil, and cook the meal on medium heat for 20 minutes. Stir the mushrooms from time to time.

per serving: 64 calories, 3.9g protein, 5.6g carbohydrates, 4g fat, 1.6g fiber, 0mg cholesterol, 8mg sodium, 423mg potassium.

Clove Artichokes

Prep time: 10 minutes | **Servings:** 4
Cook time: 25 minutes

- 4 artichokes, trimmed and halved
- 4 tablespoons avocado oil
- 1 tablespoon garlic powder
- 1 tablespoon ground clove

1. Rub the artichokes with garlic powder and ground clove. Sprinkle them with avocado oil.
2. Put the artichokes in the oven and bake at 365F for 25 minutes.

per serving: 107 calories, 5.9g protein, 20.4g carbohydrates, 2.4g fat, 10.1g fiber, 0mg cholesterol, 157mg sodium, 685mg potassium.

Sweet Quinoa

Prep time: 10 minutes | **Servings:** 4
Cook time: 20 minutes

- 1 cup pears, chopped
- 1 cup quinoa
- 3 cups of water
- 1 tablespoon almond butter

1. Mix water with quinoa and cook it on low heat for 10 minutes.
2. Then add pears and almond butter. Stir the meal and cook it for 10 minutes.

per serving: 209 calories, 7.3g protein, 34.8g carbohydrates, 5g fat, 5g fiber, 0mg cholesterol, 40mg sodium, 316mg potassium.

Cilantro Brussels Sprouts

Prep time: 10 minutes | **Servings:** 4
Cook time: 20 minutes

- 2 tablespoons olive oil
- 1 pound Brussels sprouts, trimmed and halved
- ¼ cup fresh cilantro, chopped
- 1 tablespoon lemon juice

1. Line the baking tray with baking paper.
2. Then mix Brussel sprouts with cilantro, lemon juice, and olive oil.
3. Put the vegetables in the tray in one layer and bake at 385F for 20 minutes.

per serving: 110 calories, 3.9g protein, 10.4g carbohydrates, 7.4g fat, 4.3g fiber, 0mg cholesterol, 30mg sodium, 451mg potassium.

Cauliflower Puree

Prep time: 10 minutes | **Servings:** 4
Cook time: 25 minutes

- 1 pound cauliflower florets
- 1 cup coconut cream
- 1 oz Parmesan, grated

1. Mix cauliflower with coconut cream and simmer the mixture for 10 minutes.
2. Then mash it with the help of the potato masher and mix it with parmesan.

per serving: 189 calories, 5.9g protein, 9.6g carbohydrates, 15.9g fat, 4.2g fiber, 5mg cholesterol, 109mg sodium, 501mg potassium.

Cayenne Pepper Green Beans

Prep time: 10 minutes | **Servings:** 4
Cook time: 20 minutes

- 1 teaspoon cayenne pepper
- 1 pound green beans, trimmed and halved
- 1 tablespoon avocado oil
- 2 cups of water

1. Bring the water to boil and add green beans. Cook them for 10 minutes.
2. Then remove water and add avocado oil and cayenne pepper.
3. Roast the vegetables for 2-3 minutes on high heat.

per serving: 41 calories, 2.2g protein, 8.5g carbohydrates, 0.7g fat, 4.1g fiber, 0mg cholesterol, 11mg sodium, 258mg potassium.

Lime Brussels Sprouts

Prep time: 10 minutes | **Servings:** 4
Cook time: 20 minutes

- 2 pounds Brussels sprouts, trimmed and halved
- 1 tablespoon olive oil
- 2 tablespoons lime juice
- 1 teaspoon lime zest, grated
- 1 teaspoon ground paprika

1. Mix Brussel sprouts with olive oil, lime juice, lime zest, and ground paprika.
2. Put the vegetables in the lined with the baking paper tray and bake for 20 minutes at 365F.

per serving: 130 calories, 7.8g protein, 21g carbohydrates, 4.3g fat, 8.8g fiber, 0mg cholesterol, 57mg sodium, 895mg potassium.

Cabbage Bowl

Prep time: 10 minutes | **Servings:** 4
Cook time: 20 minutes

- 4 cups white cabbage
- 1 cup tomatoes, diced
- 2 tablespoons olive oil
- 2 cups of water
- 1 teaspoon dried parsley

1. Mix white cabbage with tomatoes in the saucepan.
2. Add water, dried parsley, and olive oil.
3. Close the lid and simmer the meal on medium heat for 20 minutes.

per serving: 86 calories, 1.3g protein, 5.8g carbohydrates, 7.2g fat, 2.3g fiber, 0mg cholesterol, 19mg sodium, 229mg potassium.

Coconut Quinoa

Prep time: 10 minutes | **Servings:** 4
Cook time: 25 minutes

- 1 cup quinoa
- 2 cups of water
- 1 cup of coconut milk
- 1 teaspoon ground turmeric

1. Mix water with quinoa and coconut milk.
2. Add ground turmeric and close cook the meal on low heat for 25 minutes.

per serving: 296 calories, 7.4g protein, 31g carbohydrates, 16.9g fat, 4.4g fiber, 0mg cholesterol, 15mg sodium, 412mg potassium.

Parmesan Asparagus

Prep time: 10 minutes | **Servings:** 4
Cook time: 15 minutes

- 3 oz Parmesan, grated
- 2 tablespoons olive oil
- 1 bunch asparagus, trimmed and halved

1. Line the baking tray with baking paper.
2. Put the asparagus in the tray in one layer and sprinkle it with Parmesan and olive oil.
3. Bake the asparagus at 385F for 15 minutes.

per serving: 142 calories, 8.3g protein, 3.4g carbohydrates, 11.6g fat, 1.4g fiber, 15mg cholesterol, 199mg sodium, 135mg potassium.

Rosemary Black Beans

Prep time: 10 minutes | **Servings:** 4
Cook time: 0 minutes

- 1 tablespoon avocado oil
- 2 cups canned black beans, drained and rinsed
- 1 tablespoon dried rosemary
- 1 tablespoon lemon juice
- 1 onion, sliced

1. Mix black beans with dried rosemary and lemon juice.
2. Add onion and avocado oil. Shake the meal well.

per serving: 350 calories, 21.4g protein, 63.9g carbohydrates, 2g fat, 15.9g fiber, 0mg cholesterol, 7mg sodium, 1502mg potassium.

Quinoa Salad

Prep time: 10 minutes | **Servings:** 4
Cook time: 0 minutes

- 2 cups quinoa, cooked
- 1 cup olives, sliced
- 1 tablespoon olive oil
- 1 cucumber, chopped

1. Mix quinoa with olives, cucumber, and olive oil.
2. Shake the salad well before serving.

per serving: 393 calories, 12.8g protein, 59.4g carbohydrates, 12.3g fat, 7.4g fiber, 0mg cholesterol, 299mg sodium, 592mg potassium.

Oregano Green Beans

Prep time: 10 minutes | **Servings:** 4
Cook time: 15 minutes

- 1 pound green beans, trimmed and halved
- 1 cup of water
- 1 tablespoon dried oregano
- 1 teaspoon chili powder
- 1 tablespoon almond butter

1. Bring the water to boil.
2. Add green beans and boil them for 10 minutes.
3. Then transfer the green beans in the bowl and add dried oregano, chili powder, and almond butter.
4. Stir the meal well.

per serving: 65 calories, 3.1g protein, 9.9g carbohydrates, 2.6g fat, 5g fiber, 0mg cholesterol, 16mg sodium, 299mg potassium.

Yam Mash

Prep time: 10 minutes | **Servings:** 4
Cook time: 25 minutes

- 1-pound yams, peeled
- ¼ cup coconut cream
- 1 tablespoon dried dill

1. Bake the yams at 365F for 25 minutes.
2. Then mash the yams and mix them with coconut cream and dried dill. Stir the meal well.

per serving: 168 calories, 2.2g protein, 32.4g carbohydrates, 3.8g fat, 4.9g fiber, 0mg cholesterol, 13mg sodium, 825mg potassium.

Soft Peas

Prep time: 10 minutes | **Servings:** 4
Cook time: 20 minutes

- 1 cup coconut cream
- 2 cups green peas
- ¼ cup fresh cilantro, chopped

1. Pour coconut cream in the saucepan.
2. Add green peas and cilantro.
3. Close the lid and cook the meal on medium heat for 20 minutes.

per serving: 197 calories, 5.3g protein, 13.8g carbohydrates, 14.6g fat, 5.1g fiber, 0mg cholesterol, 13mg sodium, 340mg potassium.

Mushroom Stew

Prep time: 10 minutes | **Servings:** 4
Cook time: 35 minutes

- 1 pound mushrooms, sliced
- 1 cup onion, chopped
- ½ cup coconut cream
- 1 teaspoon ground black pepper
- 1 tablespoon olive oil
- 1 teaspoon dried dill

1. Put all ingredients in the saucepan and gently mix.
2. Close the lid and transfer the saucepan in the oven.
3. Cook the stew at 365F for 35 minutes.

per serving: 137 calories, 4.7g protein, 8.6g carbohydrates, 1g fat, 2.6g fiber, 0mg cholesterol, 13mg sodium, 496mg potassium.

Cheesy Broccoli

Prep time: 10 minutes | **Servings:** 4
Cook time: 25 minutes

- 1 pound broccoli florets
- 3 oz Romano cheese, grated
- 1 tablespoon olive oil
- ½ teaspoon ground paprika

1. Line the baking tray with baking paper.
2. Put the broccoli florets inside and sprinkle them with olive oil and ground paprika.
3. Cook the broccoli for 20 minutes at 365F.
4. Then top the vegetables with Romano cheese and bake for 5 minutes more.

per serving: 152 calories, 10g protein, 8.4g carbohydrates, 9.6g fat, 3.1g fiber, 22mg cholesterol, 293mg sodium, 383mg potassium.

Glazed Broccoli

Prep time: 10 minutes | **Servings:** 4
Cook time: 20 minutes

- 1 tablespoon avocado oil
- 1 pound broccoli florets
- 1 tablespoon raw
- honey
- 1 tablespoon rosemary, chopped
- 1 teaspoon chili powder

1. Preheat the skillet well.
2. Add broccoli florets and sprinkle them with avocado oil.
3. Add chili powder and rosemary.
4. Roast the broccoli for 7 minutes per side.
5. Then add honey, carefully mix the vegetables and cook them for 3 minutes more.

per serving: 64 calories, 3.4g protein, 13g carbohydrates, 1.1g fat, 3.7g fiber, 0mg cholesterol, 45mg sodium, 393mg potassium.

Cinnamon Asparagus

Prep time: 10 minutes | **Servings:** 4
Cook time: 20 minutes

- 1 pound asparagus, trimmed and halved
- 1 teaspoon ground cinnamon
- 1 tablespoon olive oil
- 1 teaspoon chili flakes
- 1 teaspoon lemon zest, grated

1. Mix asparagus with all remaining ingredients and put in the baking tray.
2. Flatten the asparagus in one layer and bake at 375F for 20 minutes.

per serving: 55 calories, 2.5g protein, 5g carbohydrates, 3.7g fat, 2.7g fiber, 0mg cholesterol, 2mg sodium, 234mg potassium.

Spicy Cucumbers

Prep time: 15 minutes | **Servings:** 4
Cook time: 0 minutes

- 3 cups cucumbers, chopped
- 3 tablespoons lemon juice
- 1 tablespoon olive oil
- 1 teaspoon ground coriander
- 1 teaspoon chili powder
- 1 teaspoon dried parsley

1. Put the cucumbers in the big glass jar.
2. Add all remaining ingredients and carefully mix the mixture.
3. Leave it for at least 10 minutes to marinate.

per serving: 47 calories, 0.7g protein, 3.5g carbohydrates, 3.8g fat, 0.7g fiber, 0mg cholesterol, 11mg sodium, 143mg potassium.

Summer Salad

Prep time: 10 minutes | **Servings:** 4
Cook time: 0 minutes

- 1 pound cherry tomatoes, halved
- 2 sweet peppers, chopped
- 1 cucumber, chopped
- 2 tablespoons olive oil
- 2 garlic cloves, diced

1. Mix cherry tomatoes with sweet peppers, cucumber, and garlic cloves.
2. Add olive oil and mix the salad well.

per serving: 113 calories, 2.2g protein, 12.1g carbohydrates, 7.5g fat, 2.6g fiber, 0mg cholesterol, 9mg sodium, 497mg potassium.

Tender Quinoa

Prep time: 10 minutes | **Servings:** 4
Cook time: 30 minutes

- 1 tablespoon olive oil
- 1 cup quinoa
- 2 cups of water
- 3 tablespoons almond butter

1. Mix quinoa with olive oil and put it in the saucepan.
2. Add water and boil it for 25 minutes on low heat.
3. Then add almond butter and cook the quinoa for 5 minutes more.

per serving: 260 calories, 8.6g protein, 29.5g carbohydrates, 12.8g fat, 4.2g fiber, 0mg cholesterol, 7mg sodium, 330mg potassium.

Chickpeas Bowl

Prep time: 5 minutes | **Servings:** 4
Cook time: 0 minutes

- 2 cups canned chickpeas, drained and rinsed
- 1 tomato, chopped
- 1 cup fresh cilantro, chopped
- 1 tablespoon olive oil
- 2 garlic cloves, sliced
- 2 tablespoons lemon juice

1. Mix chickpeas with tomatoes, cilantro, olive oil, garlic, and lemon juice.
2. Stir the mixture well and divide into serving bowls.

per serving: 402 calories, 19.7g protein, 62.1g carbohydrates, 9.7g fat, 17.8g fiber, 0mg cholesterol, 28mg sodium, 948mg potassium.

Beans Mash

Prep time: 10 minutes | **Servings:** 4
Cook time: 0 minutes

- 16 oz white beans, boiled
- 1 tablespoon almond butter
- ¼ cup coconut cream
- ½ teaspoon ground clove

1. Put the white beans in the blender.
2. Add almond butter, coconut cream, and ground clove.
3. Blend the mixture until smooth and transfer into the serving bowls.

per serving: 437 calories, 27.7g protein, 70.1g carbohydrates, 6.8g fat, 18.1g fiber, mg cholesterol, 21mg sodium, 2108mg potassium.

Spiralized Carrot

Prep time: 5 minutes | **Servings:** 4
Cook time: 5 minutes

- 7 carrots, spiralized
- 2 tablespoons lime juice
- 1 tablespoon olive oil
- 1 teaspoon ground black pepper

1. Preheat the olive oil in the skillet well.
2. Add carrot and ground black pepper.
3. Roast the carrot for 2-3 minutes.
4. Add lime juice, stir the carrot, and cook it for 2 minutes more.

per serving: 77 calories, 1g protein, 11.4g carbohydrates, 3.5g fat, 2.8g fiber, 0mg cholesterol, 75mg sodium, 354mg potassium.

Classic Barley

Prep time: 5 minutes | **Servings:** 4
Cook time: 30 minutes

- 2 cups barley
- 4 cups of water
- 1 tablespoon olive oil

1. Mix water with barley and olive oil.
2. Cook the barley with the closed lid for 30 minutes on low heat.

per serving: 356 calories, 11.5g protein, 67.6g carbohydrates, 5.6g fat, 15.9g fiber, 0mg cholesterol, 18mg sodium, 418mg potassium.

Baked Mango

Prep time: 5 minutes | **Servings:** 4
Cook time: 20 minutes

- 2 mangos, peeled and chopped
- 1 tablespoon
- Italian seasonings
- 1 tablespoon olive oil

1. Mix mango with Italian seasonings and olive oil.
2. Put the mango in the tray and bake it for 20 minutes at 355F.

per serving: 131 calories, 1.4g protein, 25.2g carbohydrates, 4.1g fat, 2.7g fiber, 0mg cholesterol, 2mg sodium, 282mg potassium.

Easy Cabbage Slaw

Prep time: 10 minutes | **Servings:** 4
Cook time: 0 minutes

- 2 cups green cabbage, shredded
- 1 carrot, grated
- 3 tablespoons raisins, chopped
- 2 tablespoons
- coconut cream
- 1 tablespoon lemon juice
- 1 tablespoon olive oil

1. Mix green cabbage with carrot, raisins, coconut cream, and lemon juice.
2. Then add olive oil and carefully mix the slaw.

per serving: 83 calories, 1g protein, 9.4g carbohydrates, 5.4g fat, 1.7g fiber, 0mg cholesterol, 19mg sodium, 184mg potassium.

Corn Mix

Prep time: 10 minutes | **Servings:** 4
Cook time: 0 minutes

- 1 cup corn kernels, cooked
- 1 avocado, peeled, pitted and cubed
- 2 cups arugula,
- chopped
- 1 tomato, chopped
- 1 tablespoon olive oil

1. Mix corn kernels with avocado, arugula, and tomato.
2. Then sprinkle the ingredients with olive oil and gently shake.

per serving: 171 calories, 2.6g protein, 12.5g carbohydrates, 13.9g fat, 4.8g fiber, 0mg cholesterol, 12mg sodium, 421mg potassium.

Apple Salad

Prep time: 5 minutes | **Servings:** 4
Cook time: 0 minutes

- 5 apples, chopped
- ½ cup fresh dill, chopped
- 1 tablespoon olive oil
- 1 tomato, chopped

1. Mix apples with dill and tomato.
2. Add olive oil and stir the salad one more time.

per serving: 193 calories, 2.1g protein, 42.5g carbohydrates, 4.3g fat, 7.8g fiber, 0mg cholesterol, 16mg sodium, 533mg potassium.

Avocado Mash

Prep time: 10 minutes | **Servings:** 4
Cook time: 0 minutes

- 1 tablespoon fresh cilantro, chopped
- 2 avocados, peeled, pitted and sliced
- 1 tablespoon minced garlic
- 2 tablespoons lemon juice
- 1 tablespoon olive oil

1. Blend the avocado until smooth and transfer it in the bowl.
2. Add cilantro, minced garlic, lemon juice, and olive oil.
3. Stir the meal well.

per serving: 240 calories, 2.1g protein, 9.5g carbohydrates, 23.2g fat, 6.8g fiber, 0mg cholesterol, 8mg sodium, 507mg potassium.

Bake Endives

Prep time: 10 minutes | **Servings:** 4
Cook time: 20 minutes

- 1-pound endives, roughly chopped
- 1 tablespoon olive
- oil
- 1 tablespoon garlic powder

1. Put the endives in the baking tray.
2. Sprinkle the vegetables with olive oil and garlic powder.
3. Bake the endives at 365F for 20 minutes.

per serving: 56 calories, 1.8g protein, 5.3g carbohydrates, 3.8g fat, 3.7g fiber, 0mg cholesterol, 26mg sodium, 379mg potassium.

Arugula Bowl

Prep time: 5 minutes | **Servings:** 4
Cook time: 0 minutes

- 2 cups baby arugula
- Juice of 1 lime
- 1 cup tomatoes, chopped
- 3 oz Romano cheese, crumbled
- 1 tablespoon olive oil

1. Put all ingredients in the bowl.
2. Shake the meal before serving.

per serving: 128 calories, 7.7g protein, 4.6g carbohydrates, 9.4g fat, 1.2g fiber, 22mg cholesterol, 260mg sodium, 181mg potassium.

Baked Tomatoes

Prep time: 10 minutes | **Servings:** 4
Cook time: 15 minutes

- 1-pound tomatoes, halved
- 2 tablespoons olive
- oil
- 1 tablespoon dried oregano

1. Put the tomatoes in the tray in one layer.
2. Sprinkle them with olive oil and dried oregano.
3. Bake the tomatoes at 375F for 15 minutes.

per serving: 84 calories, 1.1g protein, 5.1g carbohydrates, 7.4g fat, 1.8g fiber, 0mg cholesterol, 6mg sodium, 288mg potassium.

Baked Radish

Prep time: 10 minutes | **Servings:** 4
Cook time: 25 minutes

- 4 cups radish, halved
- 2 tablespoons olive
- oil
- 1 teaspoon dried rosemary

1. Mix radish with olive oil and dried rosemary.
2. Put the vegetables in the tray, flatten them gently and bake at 365F for 25 minutes.

per serving: 80 calories, 0.8g protein, 4.1g carbohydrates, 7.2g fat, 2g fiber, 0mg cholesterol, 45mg sodium, 273mg potassium.

Baked Okra

Prep time: 10 minutes | **Servings:** 4
Cook time: 30 minutes

- 4 cups okra, chopped
- 1 teaspoon ground clove
- 1 teaspoon cayenne pepper
- 3 tablespoons olive oil

1. Mix okra with ground clove, cayenne pepper, and olive oil.
2. Put the okra mixture in the tray and bake it at 355F for 30 minutes.

per serving: 133 calories, 2g protein, 8g carbohydrates, 10.9g fat, 3.5g fiber, 0mg cholesterol, 8mg sodium, 314mg potassium.

Baked Celery Root

Prep time: 10 minutes | **Servings:** 4
Cook time: 30 minutes

- 1-pound celery root, peeled, chopped
- 2 tablespoons olive oil
- 1 tablespoon lemon juice
- 1 teaspoon chili powder

1. Put the celery root in the tray and sprinkle with olive oil and chili powder.
2. Bake it at 365F for 30 minutes.
3. Sprinkle the cooked celery with lemon juice before serving.

per serving: 111 calories, 1.8g protein, 10.9g carbohydrates, 7.5g fat, 2.3g fiber, 0mg cholesterol, 121mg sodium, 357mg potassium.

Baked Chard

Prep time: 10 minutes | **Servings:** 4
Cook time: 15 minutes

- 1-pound swiss chard, chopped
- 1 tablespoon olive oil
- 2 oz Parmesan, grated

1. Line the baking tray with baking paper and put swiss chard inside.
2. Top it with olive oil and Parmesan and bake at 350F for 15 minutes.

per serving: 98 calories, 6.6g protein, 4.8g carbohydrates, 6.9g fat, 1.9g fiber, 10mg cholesterol, 374mg sodium, 431mg potassium.

Green Quinoa

Prep time: 10 minutes | **Servings:** 4
Cook time: 0 minutes

- 1 cup quinoa, cooked
- 2 cups spinach, blended
- 2 oz pistachios, grinded
- 2 tablespoons olive oil
- 1 oz Parmesan, grated

1. Mix spinach with pistachios, olive oil, and Parmesan.
2. Then add quinoa and carefully mix the meal.
3. Put it in the serving plates.

per serving: 318 calories, 11.5g protein, 31.9g carbohydrates, 17.8g fat, 4.7g fiber, 5mg cholesterol, 156mg sodium, 469mg potassium.

Lime Asparagus

Prep time: 10 minutes | **Servings:** 4
Cook time: 20 minutes

- 1 pound asparagus, trimmed
- 2 tablespoons olive oil
- 3 tablespoons lime juice
- 1 teaspoon lime zest, grated

1. Put the asparagus in the baking tray and sprinkle with olive oil and lime zest.
2. Bake the asparagus for 20 minutes at 360F.
3. Then sprinkle the cooked vegetables with lime juice.

per serving: 84 calories, 2.5g protein, 4.7g carbohydrates, 7.2g fat, 2.5g fiber, 0mg cholesterol, 3mg sodium, 233mg potassium.

Cabbage Steaks

Prep time: 10 minutes | **Servings:** 4
Cook time: 10 minutes

- 1-pound cabbage, sliced into steaks
- 2 tablespoons olive oil
- 1 teaspoon minced garlic

1. Rub the cabbage steaks with olive oil and minced garlic and grill in the grill at 400F for 5 minutes per side.

per serving: 89 calories, 1.5g protein, 6.8g carbohydrates, 7.1g fat, 2.9g fiber, 0mg cholesterol, 21mg sodium, 196mg potassium.

Broccoli Puree

Prep time: 10 minutes | **Servings:** 4
Cook time: 10 minutes

- 1-pound broccoli
- 2 cups of water
- ½ cup coconut
  cream
- 3 oz Parmesan,
  grated

1. Bring the water to boil and add broccoli.
2. Boil it for 10 minutes.
3. Then transfer the broccoli in the blender and blend until smooth.
4. Put the broccoli puree in the bowl, add coconut cream and Parmesan.
5. Stir the broccoli puree until smooth.

per serving: 176 calories, 10.7g protein, 10g carbohydrates, 12.1g fat, 3.6g fiber, 15mg cholesterol, 243mg sodium, 439mg potassium.

Baked Sweet Peppers

Prep time: 15 minutes | **Servings:** 4
Cook time: 20 minutes

- 4 sweet peppers,
  trimmed, seeded
- 2 tablespoons olive
  oil
- 1 tablespoon
  minced garlic
- 1 tablespoon
  lemon juice

1. Put the sweet peppers in the oven and bake them at 375F for 20 minutes.
2. When the time is over, remove the peppers from the heat and peel.
3. Chop the peppers and put them in the bowl.
4. Add olive oil, minced garlic, and lemon juice. Stir the meal.

per serving: 102 calories, 1.4g protein, 9.8g carbohydrates, 7.3g fat, 1.7g fiber, 0mg cholesterol, 4mg sodium, 237mg potassium.

Swiss Chard Mix

Prep time: 10 minutes | **Servings:** 4
Cook time: 12 minutes

- 1 pound swiss
  chard, chopped
- 1 yellow onion,
  chopped
- 1 tablespoon olive
  oil
- 1 tablespoon
  ground clove
- 2 oz Parmesan,
  grated

1. Preheat the skillet well and add olive oil. Add onion.
2. Roast it until light brown.
3. Then add Swiss chard and ground clove. Carefully mix the ingredients and cook them for 3 minutes.
4. Top the swiss chard with Parmesan and close the lid.
5. Cook the meal for 2 minutes on medium heat or until the cheese is melted.

per serving: 114 calories, 7g protein, 8.3g carbohydrates, 7.2g fat, 3g fiber, 10mg cholesterol, 379mg sodium, 489mg potassium.

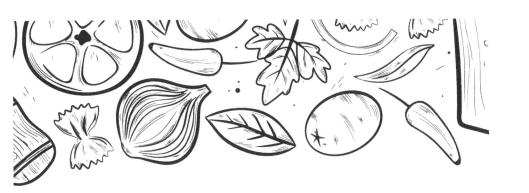

Soups

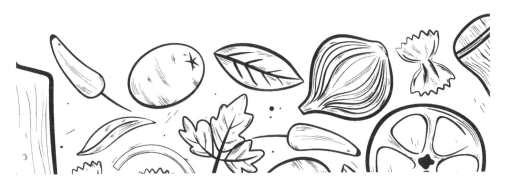

Onion Cream Soup

Prep time: 10 minutes | **Servings:** 4
Cook time: 20 minutes

- 2 cups onions, chopped
- 5 cups of water
- 1 cup sweet pepper, chopped
- 2 tablespoons olive oil
- 1 tablespoon dried dill
- 1 teaspoon ground paprika
- 2 oz Parmesan, grated

1. Mix olive oil with onions in the saucepan and roast the mixture for 5 minutes.
2. Then add water, sweet pepper, dried dill, and ground paprika.
3. Close the lid and cook the soup for 15 minutes more.
4. Then blend it with the help of the immersion blender.
5. Top the soup with Parmesan.

per serving: 142 calories, 5.7g protein, 8.9g carbohydrates, 10.3g fat, 1.9g fiber, 10mg cholesterol, 145mg sodium, 181mg potassium

Tomato Soup

Prep time: 15 minutes | **Servings:** 4
Cook time: 25 minutes

- 4 cups tomatoes, chopped
- 2 cups of water
- ½ cup fresh spinach, chopped
- 1 teaspoon garlic, diced
- 1 teaspoon ground paprika
- 1 teaspoon cayenne pepper
- 1 cup broccoli, chopped

1. Put all ingredients in the saucepan and close the lid.
2. Simmer the soup for 20 minutes on the medium heat.
3. Blend the soup with the help of the immersion blender.
4. Bring the cream soup to boil and cook for 5 minutes more.

per serving: 45 calories, 2.5g protein, 9.4g carbohydrates, 0.6g fat, 3.2g fiber, 0mg cholesterol, 23mg sodium, 545mg potassium.

Broccoli Soup

Prep time: 10 minutes | **Servings:** 4
Cook time: 35 minutes

- 1 yellow onion, chopped
- 1 carrot, chopped
- 2 cups broccoli, hopped
- 1 tablespoon olive
- oil
- 5 cups of water
- 1 cup tomatoes, chopped
- 1 teaspoon chili powder

1. Pour olive oil in the saucepan.
2. Add onion and carrot. Roast the vegetables for 5 minutes on medium heat.
3. Then add broccoli, water, tomatoes, and chili powder.
4. Close the lid and cook the soup on medium heat for 30 minutes.

per serving: 73 calories, 2.2g protein, 9.2g carbohydrates, 3.9g fat, 2.9g fiber, 0mg cholesterol, 44mg sodium, 355mg potassium.

Garlic Cream Soup

Prep time: 10 minutes | **Servings:** 4
Cook time: 30 minutes

- 3 large zucchinis, chopped
- 1 cup coconut cream
- 4 cups of water
- 1 teaspoon minced
- garlic
- 1 cup pumpkin, chopped
- 1 teaspoon pumpkin pie spices

1. Pour water in the saucepan.
2. Add pumpkin, zucchinis, and pumpkin pie spices.
3. Add minced garlic and bring the liquid to boil. Simmer the soup for 15 minutes.
4. Blend the soup until smooth and add coconut cream.
5. Bring the soup to boil and remove from the heat.

per serving: 200 calories, 5g protein, 16.9g carbohydrates, 15g fat, 5.8g fiber, 0mg cholesterol, 44mg sodium, 927mg potassium

Ginger Cauliflower Soup

Prep time: 10 minutes | **Servings:** 4
Cook time: 25 minutes

- 2 carrots, peeled and grated
- 1 pound cauliflower, chopped
- 1 teaspoon minced garlic
- 1 tablespoon olive oil
- 1 teaspoon chili powder
- 4 cups of water
- 1 teaspoon ginger, grated
- ½ cup fresh cilantro, chopped

1. Pour olive oil in the saucepan.
2. Add minced garlic, ginger, and chili powder.
3. Stir the mixture and cook it for 2 minutes.
4. Then add all remaining ingredients and carefully stir the soup with the help of the spoon.
5. Cook it for 23 minutes.

per serving: 76 calories, 2.7g protein, 10g carbohydrates, 3.8g fat, 3.9g fiber, 0mg cholesterol, 70mg sodium, 475mg potassium.

Green Soup

Prep time: 10 minutes | **Servings:** 4
Cook time: 20 minutes

- 1 pound spinach, chopped
- 1 yellow onion, chopped
- 1 tablespoon olive oil
- 4 cups of water
- 4 cherry tomatoes, halved
- ½ cup fresh cilantro, chopped

1. Pour the olive oil in the saucepan.
2. Add onions and roast them for 2-3 minutes.
3. Then add spinach, tomatoes, and fresh cilantro.
4. Close the lid and cook the soup on medium heat for 18 minutes.

per serving: 90 calories, 4.7g protein, 11.5g carbohydrates, 4.2g fat, 4.6g fiber, 0mg cholesterol, 105mg sodium, 977mg potassium.

Chicken Soup

Prep time: 10 minutes | **Servings:** 8
Cook time: 1 hour

- 1 onion, diced
- 1 cup yams, chopped
- 1-pound chicken breast, boneless, chopped
- 8 cups of water
- 1 cup fresh parsley, chopped
- 1 teaspoon dried rosemary
- 1 teaspoon ground nutmeg

1. Pour water in the saucepan.
2. Add chicken and cook it for 20 minutes.
3. Then add onion, yams, parsley, ground nutmeg, and dried rosemary.
4. Close the lid and simmer the soup on low heat for 40 minutes.

per serving: 95 calories, 12.7 g protein, 6.7g carbohydrates, 1.6g fat, 1.3g fiber, 36mg cholesterol, 42mg sodium, 390mg potassium.

Coconut Soup

Prep time: 10 minutes | **Servings:** 7
Cook time: 25 minutes

- 3 cups of coconut milk
- 4 cups of water
- 1 cup zucchini, chopped
- 1 cup broccoli, chopped
- 3 oz Romano cheese, grated
- 1 teaspoon chili powder
- 1 teaspoon dried mint

1. Pour water and coconut milk in the saucepan.
2. Add mint and chili powder.
3. Then add broccoli and cook the soup for 10 minutes.
4. After this, add zucchini and grated cheese.
5. Cook the soup for 10 minutes more.

per serving: 292 calories, 6.8g protein, 7.8g carbohydrates, 27.9g fat, 2.9g fiber, 13mg cholesterol, 175mg sodium, 374mg potassium

Shrimp Soup

Prep time: 5 minutes | **Servings:** 4
Cook time: 25 minutes

- 4 cups of water
- 1-pound shrimps, peeled
- 1 teaspoon dried rosemary
- ¼ cup Plain yogurt
- 1 teaspoon chili powder
- 1 onion, diced
- 1 teaspoon olive oil

1. Mix olive oil with onion in the saucepan and roast the mixture on medium heat until onion is light brown.
2. Then add all remaining ingredients and close the lid.
3. Cook the soup for 20 minutes on medium heat.

per serving: 170 calories, 27.1g protein, 5.9g carbohydrates, 3.5g fat, 0.9g fiber, 240mg cholesterol, 302mg sodium, 286mg potassium

Mushroom Cream Soup

Prep time: 10 minutes | **Servings:** 4
Cook time: 30 minutes

- 1-pound mushrooms, chopped
- 1 cup plain yogurt
- 4 cups of water
- 2 onions, diced
- 1 tablespoon olive oil
- 3 oz Parmesan, grated

1. Mix olive oil with mushrooms in the saucepan and roast the mixture for 5 minutes.
2. Add plain yogurt, water, onion, and simmer the soup for 20 minutes.
3. Blend the soup with the help of the immersion blender and top with Parmesan.

per serving: 188 calories, 14.5g protein, 13.9g carbohydrates, 9.2g fat, 2.3g fiber, 19mg cholesterol, 256mg sodium, 587mg potassium

Spinach Soup

Prep time: 10 minutes | **Servings:** 4
Cook time: 25 minutes

- 1 cup carrot, grated
- 2 cups spinach, chopped
- 1 onion, diced
- 1 tablespoon olive
- oil
- 1 teaspoon garlic powder
- 1 teaspoon dried dill
- 5 cups of water

1. Pour olive oil in the saucepan.
2. Add onion and roast it until light brown.
3. Add carrot, garlic powder, dried dill, and water.
4. Simmer the soup for 10 minutes.
5. Add spinach and bring the soup to boil.

per serving: 59 calories, 1.1g protein, 6.5g carbohydrates, 3.6g fat, 1.7g fiber, 0mg cholesterol, 41mg sodium, 231mg potassium

Yellow Soup

Prep time: 10 minutes | **Servings:** 4

Cook time: 25 minutes
2 cups carrot, chopped

- 1 cup pumpkin, chopped
- 1 teaspoon ground cinnamon
- 1 tablespoon
- lemon juice
- 1 teaspoon lemon zest, grated
- 6 cups of water

1. Put all ingredients in the saucepan and close the lid.
2. Cook the soup on medium heat for 25 minutes or until all ingredients are soft.

per serving: 46 calories, 1.2g protein, 11g carbohydrates, 0.2g fat, 3.5g fiber, 0mg cholesterol, 52mg sodium, 314mg potassium

Green Peas Soup

Prep time: 10 minutes | **Servings:** 6
Cook time: 35 minutes

- 1 onion, chopped
- 1 pound green peas
- 1 carrot, grated
- 6 cups of water
- 1 tablespoon dried
- sage
- 1 teaspoon cayenne pepper
- 2 tablespoons olive oil

1. Pour olive oil in the saucepan. Add carrot and roast it for 5 minutes.
2. Then add onion, green peas, sage, and cayenne pepper.
3. Close the lid and simmer the soup on low heat for 30 minutes.

per serving: 115 calories, 4.5g protein, 14g carbohydrates, 5.1g fat, 4.7g fiber, 0mg cholesterol, 19mg sodium, 256mg potassium

Red Soup

Prep time: 10 minutes | **Servings:** 6
Cook time: 30 minutes

- 2 cups cabbage, shredded
- 2 cups tomatoes, chopped
- 4 oz leek, chopped
- 6 cups of water
- 1 cup tomato juice

1. Pour water in the saucepan. Add tomatoes and bring the mixture to boil.
2. Then blend the mixture until smooth.
3. Add cabbage, leek, and tomato juice.
4. Simmer the soup for 20 minutes on low heat.

per serving: 35 calories, 1.4g protein, 8.1g carbohydrates, 0.2g fat, 1.8g fiber, 0mg cholesterol, 127mg sodium, 311mg potassium

Lentils Soup

Prep time: 10 minutes | **Servings:** 4
Cook time: 30 minutes

- 1 cup lentils
- 6 cups of water
- 1 onion, diced
- 1 chili pepper, diced
- 2 tablespoons tomato paste
- 2 tablespoons olive oil

1. Mix onion with olive oil in the saucepan and roast for 2-3 minutes.
2. Then add lentils, chili pepper, and tomato paste. Stir the mixture.
3. Add water and stir the soup again.
4. Close the lid and cook the soup for 25 minutes.

per serving: 247 calories, 13g protein, 33g carbohydrates, 7.6g fat, 15.6g fiber, 0mg cholesterol, 23mg sodium, 586mg potassium

Chard Soup

Prep time: 10 minutes | **Servings:** 4
Cook time: 25 minutes

- 2 cups coconut cream
- 2 cups of water
- 1-pound swiss chard, chopped
- 1 cup broccoli, chopped
- 1 teaspoon ground black pepper

1. Mix coconut cream with water in the saucepan.
2. Add broccoli and ground black pepper.
3. Bring the soup to boil and cook it for 10 minutes.
4. Then add Swiss chard and cook the soup for 10 minutes more.

per serving: 307 calories, 5.5g protein, 12.7g carbohydrates, 29g fat, 5.3g fiber, 0mg cholesterol, 272mg sodium, 826mg potassium

Zoodle Soup

Prep time: 10 minutes | **Servings:** 4
Cook time: 25 minutes

- 3 zucchinis, spiralized
- 1 cup coconut cream
- 3 cups of water
- 1 tablespoon dried parsley
- 1 teaspoon dried dill
- 1 teaspoon dried oregano
- 1 teaspoon olive oil

1. Pour the olive oil in the saucepan.
2. Add dried parsley, dill, and oregano. Stir the mixture.
3. Add water and coconut cream.
4. When the liquid starts to boil, add spiralized zucchinis and boil it for 5 minutes.

per serving: 174 calories, 3.3g protein, 8.7g carbohydrates, 15.8g fat, 3.2g fiber, 0mg cholesterol, 30mg sodium, 565mg potassium

Meatball Soup

Prep time: 10 minutes | **Servings:** 4
Cook time: 30 minutes

2 cups ground chicken

- 1 teaspoon chili powder
- 5 cups of water
- 1 onion, diced
- 1 tablespoon olive oil
- 2 carrots, grated

1. Mix ground chicken with chili powder. Make the meatballs.
2. Pour water in the saucepan.
3. Add onion, olive oil, and carrot.
4. Bring the soup to boil and add meatballs.
5. Close the lid and cook the soup on medium heat for 20 minutes.

per serving: 189 calories, 20.9g protein, 5.9g carbohydrates, 8.8g fat, 1.6g fiber, 62mg cholesterol, 98mg sodium, 323mg potassium

Tropical Soup

Prep time: 10 minutes | **Servings:** 4
Cook time: 10 minutes

- 2 avocados, pitted, peeled, chopped
- 4 cups chicken stock
- 1 teaspoon
- lemongrass, chopped
- 2 oz chives, chopped

1. Bring the chicken stock to boil.
2. Add lemongrass and chives.
3. Then add avocados and remove the soup from heat.
4. Let the soup rest for 5-10 minutes before serving.

per serving: 219 calories, 3.1g protein, 10.1g carbohydrates, 20.3g fat, 7.1g fiber, 0mg cholesterol, 770mg sodium, 547mg potassium

Yam Soup

Prep time: 10 minutes | **Servings:** 4
Cook time: 35 minutes

- 1 onion, diced
- 1 tablespoon sunflower oil
- 2 cups yams,
- chopped
- 5 cups of water
- 1 chili pepper, chopped

1. Mix onion with sunflower oil in the saucepan. Roast the mixture for 2-3 minutes.
2. Then add yams and chili pepper.
3. Add water and close the lid.
4. Cook the soup on medium heat for 30 minutes.

per serving: 121 calories, 1.3g protein, 21.4g carbohydrates, 3.6g fat, 3.3g fiber, 0mg cholesterol, 16mg sodium, 501mg potassium

Cumin Soup

Prep time: 10 minutes | **Servings:** 4
Cook time: 30 minutes

- 1 teaspoon cumin seeds
- 5 cups of water
- 1–pound salmon fillet, chopped
- 1 teaspoon olive oil
- 2 oz chives, chopped
- 1 carrot, grated

1. Mix olive oil with cumin seeds in the saucepan and roast the mixture for 5 minutes on medium heat.
2. Then add all remaining ingredients. Gently mix the mixture.
3. Close the lid and cook the soup on medium heat for 25 minutes.

per serving: 172 calories, 22.7g protein, 2.4g carbohydrates, 8.4g fat, 0.8g fiber, 50mg cholesterol, 71mg sodium, 539mg potassium

Turmeric Soup

Prep time: 10 minutes | **Servings:** 2
Cook time: 25 minutes

- ½ cup parsnip, chopped
- 1 teaspoon ground turmeric
- 1 teaspoon ground coriander
- 1 teaspoon dried rosemary
- 1 cup plain yogurt
- 2 cups of water
- 1 sweet pepper, chopped

1. Put all ingredients in the saucepan and gently mix.
2. Close the lid and cook the soup on medium heat for 25 minutes.

per serving: 137 calories, 8.1g protein, 20.2g carbohydrates, 2g fat, 2.9g fiber, 7mg cholesterol, 99mg sodium, 560mg potassium

Crab Soup

Prep time: 10 minutes | **Servings:** 6
Cook time: 20 minutes

- 1-pound crab meat, chopped
- 1 cup of coconut milk
- ½ cup fresh cilantro, chopped
- 1 cup zucchini, chopped
- 1 teaspoon cayenne pepper
- 1 tablespoon olive oil

1. Mix zucchini with olive oil in the saucepan. Roast the vegetables for 2-3 minutes per side.
2. Then add cayenne pepper and crab meat. Stir the ingredients.
3. Add cilantro and coconut milk.
4. Cook the soup for 10 minutes more.

per serving: 184 calories, 10.7g protein, 4.4g carbohydrates, 13.3g fat, 1.2g fiber, 41mg cholesterol, 481mg sodium, 168mg potassium

Ground Soup

Prep time: 10 minutes | **Servings:** 4
Cook time: 25 minutes

- 4 cups of water
- 1 cup ground chicken
- 1 cup leek, chopped
- 1 tablespoon olive
- oil
- 1 teaspoon ground coriander
- 1 teaspoon dried oregano

1. Mix olive oil with leek in the saucepan. Roast the mixture for 5 minutes.
2. Add ground chicken, ground coriander, and dried oregano.
3. Then add water and stir the soup.
4. Cook it with the closed lid for 15 minutes on medium heat.

per serving: 111 calories, 10.5g protein, 3.4g carbohydrates, 6.2g fat, 0.6g fiber, 31mg cholesterol, 42mg sodium, 134mg potassium

Cauliflower Cream Soup

Prep time: 10 minutes | **Servings:** 4
Cook time: 25 minutes

- 2 cups cauliflower, chopped
- 4 cups of water
- 1 cup coconut cream
- ½ cup fresh dill, chopped
- 1 teaspoon ground clove
- 1 teaspoon onion powder
- 1 oz Parmesan, grated

1. Put all ingredients except Parmesan in the saucepan.
2. Close the lid and simmer the soup for 20 minutes.
3. Then blend it with the help of the immersion blender.
4. When the mixture is smooth, bring it to boil one more time.
5. Ladle the soup in the serving bowls and top with Parmesan.

per serving: 192 calories, 5.9g protein, 10.4g carbohydrates, 16.3g fat, 3.6g fiber, 5mg cholesterol, 111mg sodium, 522mg potassium

Bean Soup

Prep time: 10 minutes | **Servings:** 6
Cook time: 25 minutes

- 1 cup tomatoes, chopped
- 1 cup white beans, cooked
- 6 cups of water
- 1 teaspoon ground
- black pepper
- 1 teaspoon ground paprika
- 1 onion, diced
- 1 tablespoon olive oil

1. Pour olive oil in the saucepan.
2. Add onion and tomatoes. Roast the ingredients for 5 minutes.
3. Add white beans, ground black pepper, and paprika.
4. Stir the soup and cook it for 15 minutes on medium heat.

per serving: 147 calories, 8.4g protein, 23.6g carbohydrates, 2.8g fat, 6.1g fiber, 0mg cholesterol, 15mg sodium, 717mg potassium

Seafood Soup

Prep time: 10 minutes | **Servings:** 4
Cook time: 20 minutes

- 1-pound mussels
- 1 cup tomatoes, chopped
- 2 teaspoons minced garlic
- ½ cup fresh cilantro, chopped
- 5 cups of water
- 1 teaspoon chili pepper

1. Put tomatoes, minced garlic, and water in the saucepan.
2. Add chili pepper and bring the mixture to boil.
3. Add mussels and fresh cilantro.
4. Simmer the soup for 10 minutes.

per serving: 109 calories, 14g protein, 6.6g carbohydrates, 2.7g fat, 0.7g fiber, 32mg cholesterol, 337mg sodium, 492mg potassium

Rosemary Soup

Prep time: 10 minutes | **Servings:** 6
Cook time: 35 minutes

- 6 cups of water
- 1-pound chicken breast, skinless, boneless, chopped
- 1 teaspoon dried rosemary
- 1 teaspoon dried dill
- 1 garlic clove, diced

1. Put all ingredients in the saucepan.
2. Close the lid and bring the mixture to boil.
3. Cook the soup on medium heat for 30 minutes.

per serving: 88 calories, 16.1g protein, 0.4g carbohydrates, 1.9g fat, 0.1g fiber, 48mg cholesterol, 46mg sodium, 292mg potassium

Barley Soup

Prep time: 10 minutes | **Servings:** 4
Cook time: 30 minutes

- ½ cup barley, cooked
- 5 cups of water
- 1 cup broccoli, chopped
- 1 teaspoon chili powder
- 1 teaspoon ground coriander
- 1 teaspoon cayenne pepper
- 1 onion, diced

1. Put all ingredients in the saucepan and stir gently.
2. Close the lid and cook the soup on medium heat for 30 minutes.

per serving: 104 calories, 3.9g protein, 21.6g carbohydrates, 0.8g fat, 5.5g fiber, 0mg cholesterol, 27mg sodium, 241mg potassium

Sweet Potato Soup

Prep time: 10 minutes | **Servings:** 4
Cook time: 30 minutes

- 1 teaspoon ground cinnamon
- ½ teaspoon ground ginger
- 1 teaspoon ground turmeric
- 1 teaspoon ground paprika
- 2 cups sweet potato, chopped
- 5 cups of water
- ¼ cup plain yogurt

1. In the shallow bowl, mix ground cinnamon, ground ginger, turmeric, and paprika.
2. Then Pour water in the saucepan. Add sweet potato and cook it for 20 minutes.
3. After this, add plain yogurt and spice mixture.
4. Stir the soup and boil it for 10 minutes.

per serving: 107 calories, 3.1g protein, 23.1g carbohydrates, 0.5g fat, 4g fiber, 1mg cholesterol, 56mg sodium, 546mg potassium

Beet Soup

Prep time: 10 minutes | **Servings:** 4
Cook time: 35 minutes

- 7 oz beets, peeled, chopped
- 1 cup cauliflower, chopped
- 1 oz chives, chopped
- 5 cups of water
- 1 tablespoon olive oil
- 1 teaspoon ground coriander
- ¼ cup fresh dill, chopped

1. Mix beets with olive oil in the saucepan. Roast the beets for 2 minutes per side.
2. Then add cauliflower, ground coriander, and water.
3. Bring the mixture to boil.
4. Add chives and dill. Cook the soup for 20 minutes more.

per serving: 68 calories, 2.2g protein, 8.3g carbohydrates, 3.8g fat, 2.2g fiber, 0mg cholesterol, 61mg sodium, 351mg potassium

Asparagus Soup

Prep time: 10 minutes | **Servings:** 2
Cook time: 35 minutes

- 1 cup mushrooms, chopped
- 1 cup coconut cream
- 8 oz asparagus, chopped
- 1 tablespoon avocado oil
- 2 cups of water
- 1 teaspoon cayenne pepper

1. Mix mushrooms with avocado oil in the saucepan. Roast the vegetables for 6 minutes.
2. Then add coconut cream, asparagus, water, and cayenne pepper. Stir the mixture well.
3. Cook the soup for 25 minutes.

per serving: 318 calories, 6.5g protein, 13.1g carbohydrates, 29.9g fat, 5.9g fiber, 0mg cholesterol, 30mg sodium, 699mg potassium

Oatmeal Soup

Prep time: 10 minutes | **Servings:** 2
Cook time: 25 minutes

- ½ cup plain yogurt
- 2 cups of water
- 1 cup oatmeal
- 1 zucchini, chopped
- 1 tablespoon olive oil
- 1 teaspoon chili flakes

1. Mix plain yogurt with water in the saucepan and bring the mixture to boil.
2. Add zucchini, olive oil, and chili flakes.
3. Bring the soup to boil and add oatmeal.
4. Bring the soup to boil and cook for 10 minutes on high heat.

per serving: 275 calories, 10.1g protein, 35.3g carbohydrates, 10.6g fat, 5.2g fiber, 4mg cholesterol, 62mg sodium, 553mg potassium

Celery Cream Soup

Prep time: 10 minutes | **Servings:** 2
Cook time: 25 minutes

- 12 oz celery root, peeled, chopped
- 2 cups of water
- ½ cup fresh parsley
- 2 oz Parmesan, grated
- 2 tablespoons plain yogurt
- 1 teaspoon chili powder

1. Bring the water to boil.
2. Add celery root, chili powder, and plain yogurt.
3. Bring the mixture to boil.
4. Add parsley and cook the soup for 15 minutes.
5. Ladle the soup in the bowls and top it with Parmesan.

per serving: 183 calories, 13.1g protein, 19.4g carbohydrates, 7.1g fat, 4g fiber, 21mg cholesterol, 473mg sodium, 657mg potassium

Modern Gazpacho

Prep time: 25 minutes | **Servings:** 4
Cook time: 0 minutes

- 2 cup grapes, chopped
- 1 teaspoon olive oil
- 2 cups of coconut milk
- 1 cucumber, chopped
- 1 teaspoon ground black pepper

1. Put all ingredients in the blender and blend them gently.
2. Pour the mixture in the bowls and refrigerate for 10-15 minutes before serving.

per serving: 329 calories, 3.6g protein, 17.6g carbohydrates, 30g fat, 3.6g fiber, 0mg cholesterol, 21mg sodium, 521mg potassium

Chickpea Soup

Prep time: 10 minutes | **Servings:** 4
Cook time: 30 minutes

- 1 cup plain yogurt
- 1 tablespoon Italian seasonings
- 1 cup chickpeas, cooked
- 3 cups of water
- ½ cup onion, chopped

1. Put all ingredients in the saucepan and carefully stir.
2. Close the lid and cook the soup on the medium heat for 30 minutes.

per serving: 242 calories, 13.3g protein, 36.4g carbohydrates, 4.8g fat, 9g fiber, 6mg cholesterol, 62mg sodium, 605mg potassium

Sweet Soup

Prep time: 10 minutes | **Servings:** 3
Cook time: 30 minutes

- 1 cup pumpkin, chopped
- 3 cups tomatoes, chopped
- 1 cup of water
- 1 teaspoon ground nutmeg
- 1 teaspoon olive oil

1. Mix pumpkin with olive oil and roast for 2-3 minutes per side.
2. Then put the pumpkin in the saucepan.
3. Add tomatoes, water, and ground nutmeg.
4. Cook the soup for 20 minutes on medium heat.
5. Then blend it until smooth with the help of the immersion blender.
6. Ladle the cooked soup in the bowls.

per serving: 77 calories, 2.5g protein, 14g carbohydrates, 2.4g fat, 4.7g fiber, 0mg cholesterol, 15mg sodium, 598mg potassium

Parsnip Cream Soup

Prep time: 10 minutes | **Servings:** 4
Cook time: 35 minutes

- 3 cups parsnip, chopped
- 1 cup cauliflower, chopped
- 1 teaspoon minced garlic
- 1 teaspoon dried dill
- 4 cups of water
- 1 teaspoon ground clove
- 1 tablespoon olive oil

1. Mix cauliflower with olive oil and roast it for 2 minutes per side.
2. Then put the cauliflower in the saucepan. Add parsnip, minced garlic, and dried dill.
3. Add water and ground clove.
4. Cook the soup for 30 minutes on low heat.
5. When all ingredients of the soup are soft, blend the soup with the help of immersion blender.
6. When the soup is smooth, it is cooked.

per serving: 114 calories, 1.8g protein, 20g carbohydrates, 4g fat, 5.7g fiber, 0mg cholesterol, 27mg sodium, 469mg potassium

Wedges Soup

Prep time: 10 minutes | **Servings:** 4
Cook time: 15 minutes

- 1 sweet pepper
- 1 zucchini
- 1 eggplant
- 1 tablespoon olive oil
- 1 teaspoon cayenne pepper
- 2 tablespoons plain yogurt
- 4 cups of water

1. Cut eggplant, zucchini, and sweet pepper into the wedges.
2. Then put all vegetables in the saucepan and sprinkle with olive oil.
3. Roast the vegetables for 5 minutes.
4. Then stir them well and add cayenne pepper, plain yogurt, and water. Stir the mixture.
5. Close the lid and cook the soup for 10 minutes on medium heat.

per serving: 83 calories, 2.5g protein, 11.4g carbohydrates, 4.1g fat, 5.1g fiber, 0mg cholesterol, 21mg sodium, 476mg potassium

Sorrel Soup

Prep time: 10 minutes | **Servings:** 8
Cook time: 30 minutes

- 8 cups of water
- 4 cups tomatoes, chopped
- 2 cups sorrel, chopped
- 1 cup spinach, chopped
- 2 cups cauliflower, chopped
- 1 onion, chopped
- 1 tablespoon avocado oil
- 1 teaspoon dried basil

1. Pour olive oil in the saucepan. Add onion and roast it for 3-4 minutes on medium heat.
2. Then add dried basil, cauliflower, and tomatoes.
3. Add water and cook the soup for 10 minutes.
4. After this, add sorrel and cook the soup for 16 minutes more.
5. Let the soup rest before serving.

per serving: 38 calories, 2.2g protein, 7.4g carbohydrates, 0.7g fat, 3.1g fiber, 0mg cholesterol, 24mg sodium, 468mg potassium

Taco Soup

Prep time: 10 minutes | **Servings:** 4
Cook time: 30 minutes

- 1-pound chicken fillet, chopped
- 1 tablespoon taco seasonings
- 1 cup kale, chopped
- ¼ cup of brown rice
- 5 cups of water

1. Pour water in the saucepan. Add brown rice and chicken fillet, and cook the ingredients for 20 minutes.
2. After this, add taco seasonings and kale. Stir the soup and cook it for 10 minutes more.

per serving: 274 calories, 34.2g protein, 12.3g carbohydrates, 8.7g fat, 0.7g fiber, 101mg cholesterol, 272mg sodium, 393mg potassium

Lunch Soup

Prep time: 10 minutes | **Servings:** 4
Cook time: 25 minutes

- 1-pound chicken fillet, chopped
- 4 cups of water
- 2 oz chives, chopped
- 1 teaspoon ground paprika
- 1 zucchini, chopped

1. Mix water with chicken fillet in the saucepan.
2. Bring the mixture to boil.
3. Add ground paprika and chives. Simmer the ingredients for 10 minutes.
4. Then add chopped zucchini and cook the soup for 10 minutes more.

per serving: 229 calories, 33.9g protein, 2.6g carbohydrates, 8.7g fat, 1.1g fiber, 101mg cholesterol, 110mg sodium, 461mg potassium

Rice Soup

Prep time: 10 minutes | **Servings:** 4
Cook time: 30 minutes

- 1 cup pepper, chopped
- ½ cup of brown rice
- 6 cups of water
- ½ cup plain yogurt
- 1 teaspoon dried basil
- ½ teaspoon ground nutmeg

1. Pour water in the saucepan.
2. Add brown rice and cook it for 15 minutes.
3. Then add pepper, plain yogurt, dried basil, and ground nutmeg.
4. Cook the soup for 15 minutes more.

per serving: 134 calories, 4.6g protein, 26.6g carbohydrates, 1.4g fat, 3.4g fiber, 2mg cholesterol, 37mg sodium, 261mg potassium

Dill Soup

Prep time: 10 minutes | **Servings:** 8
Cook time: 45 minutes

- 1 cup fresh dill, chopped
- 8 cups of water
- 1-pound pork tenderloin,
- chopped
- 2 onions, diced
- 1 teaspoon cumin seeds

1. Mix water with pork tenderloin and cook the ingredients for 25 minutes on medium heat.
2. Then add onion, cumin seeds, and dill.
3. Cook the soup for 20 minutes more.

per serving: 108 calories, 16.4g protein, 6g carbohydrates, 2.3g fat, 1.4g fiber, 41mg cholesterol, 53mg sodium, 484mg potassium

Wild Rice Soup

Prep time: 10 minutes | **Servings:** 4
Cook time: 35 minutes

- ½ cup wild rice
- 5 cups of water
- 1-pound chicken fillet, chopped
- 1 teaspoon dried
- basil
- 1 teaspoon ground turmeric
- 1 teaspoon olive oil

4. Mix water with wild rice and cook the mixture for 15 minutes on medium heat.
5. Then add chicken fillet and dried basil.
6. Add ground turmeric and olive oil.
7. Cook the soup for 20 minutes more.

per serving: 299 calories, 35.8g protein, 15.4g carbohydrates, 9.8g fat, 1.4g fiber, 101mg cholesterol, 108mg sodium, 378mg potassium

Cold Soup

Prep time: 40 minutes | **Servings:** 2
Cook time: 0 minutes

- 1 teaspoon ground clove
- 1 cup apples, chopped
- 1 cup pears, chopped
- 1 mango, pitted, chopped
- ½ cup of water
- 1 cup fresh spinach, chopped
- Ice cubes

1. Put all ingredients in the blender and carefully blend.
2. Then place the soup in the fridge for 30 minutes.
3. Ladle the cold soup in the bowls and add ice cubes.

per serving: 212 calories, 2.5g protein, 54g carbohydrates, 1.2g fat, 8.6g fiber, 0mg cholesterol, 20mg sodium, 591mg potassium

Corn Soup

Prep time: 10 minutes | **Servings:** 6
Cook time: 20 minutes

- 5 cups of water
- 2 cups corn kernels
- 1 cup green peas
- 12 oz chicken fillet, chopped
- 1 teaspoon fresh parsley, chopped
- 1 teaspoon ground paprika
- ½ teaspoon cayenne pepper

1. Put all ingredients in the saucepan and gently mix.
2. Close the lid and simmer the soup on medium heat for 20 minutes.

per serving: 173 calories, 19.5g protein, 13.5g carbohydrates, 5g fat, 2.8g fiber, 50mg cholesterol, 64mg sodium, 350mg potassium

Spring Soup

Prep time: 10 minutes | **Servings:** 4
Cook time: 20 minutes

- 1 cup of coconut milk
- 4 cups of water
- 1 cup sorrel, chopped
- 1 cup spinach, chopped
- 1 cup zucchini, chopped
- 1 tablespoon olive oil
- 1 chili pepper, chopped

1. Mix coconut milk with water and pour the liquid in the saucepan.
2. Add spinach, zucchini, olive oil, chili pepper, and sorrel.
3. Stir the ingredients carefully and close the lid.
4. Cook the soup on medium heat for 20 minutes.

per serving: 91 calories, 1.3g protein, 2.8g carbohydrates, 9.1g fat, 1.4g fiber, 0mg cholesterol, 13mg sodium, 204mg potassium

Curry Soup

Prep time: 10 minutes | **Servings:** 4
Cook time: 25 minutes

- 1 tablespoon curry paste
- 4 cup of water
- 1 cup of coconut milk
- 1-pound cod,
- chopped
- 1 cup onion, chopped
- 1 tablespoon olive oil

1. Mix curry paste with coconut milk.
2. Then pour olive oil in the saucepan.
3. Add onion and roast it for 2 minutes per side.
4. Add coconut milk mixture, water, and cod.
5. Stir the soup gently and cook it with the closed lid for 20 minutes.

per serving: 324 calories, 27.8g protein, 7.1g carbohydrates, 21g fat, 1.9g fiber, 62mg cholesterol, 106mg sodium, 479mg potassium

Spicy Winter Soup

Prep time: 10 minutes | **Servings:** 4
Cook time: 30 minutes

- 1 teaspoon ground cinnamon
- 1 teaspoon minced ginger
- 1 cup coconut
- cream
- 4 cups of water
- 3 cups pumpkin, chopped

1. Put all ingredients in the saucepan and cook it on medium heat for 30 minutes.
2. Then blend the soup until smooth and bring it to boil.
3. Ladle the hot soup in the bowls.

per serving: 203 calories, 3.5g protein, 19g carbohydrates, 14.9g fat, 7g fiber, 0mg cholesterol, 26mg sodium, 547mg potassium

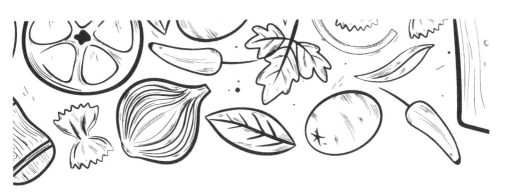

Salads

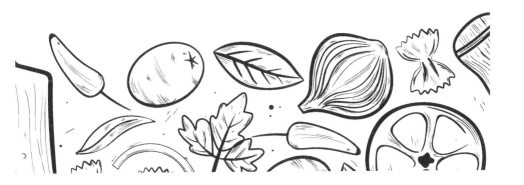

Peach Salad

Prep time: 5 minutes | **Cook time:** 0 minutes | **Servings:** 4

- 1 cup lettuce, chopped
- 1 tablespoon scallions, chopped
- 1 teaspoon minced garlic
- 1 tablespoon olive oil
- 2 cups peaches, chopped
- 12 oz cod fillet, boiled, chopped
- 1 tablespoon lime juice

1. Mix lettuce with scallions, minced garlic, peaches, and cod fillet.
2. Put the salad in the serving plates and sprinkle it with lime juice and olive oil.

per serving: 132 calories, 16g protein, 8g carbohydrates, 4.5g fat, 1.3g fiber, 42mg cholesterol, 55mg sodium, 42mg potassium

Pineapple Salad

Prep time: 10 minutes | **Cook time:** 0 minutes | **Servings:** 4

- 10 oz pineapple, chopped
- 1 mango, chopped
- 1 tablespoon coconut cream
- 1 teaspoon lemon juice
- 1 tablespoon coconut shred

1. Mix pineapple with mango, and coconut shred.
2. Then sprinkle the salad with coconut cream and lemon juice.

per serving: 107 calories, 1.2g protein, 22.6g carbohydrates, 2.6g fat, 2.7g fiber, 0mg cholesterol, 3mg sodium, 230mg potassium

Nutmeg Tomato Salad

Prep time: 5 minutes | **Cook time:** 0 minutes | **Servings:** 4

- 7 tomatoes, chopped
- 1 teaspoon ground nutmeg
- 3 garlic cloves, diced
- 1 tablespoon olive oil
- 1 teaspoon lemon juice
- ½ cup fresh dill, chopped

1. Put all ingredients in the salad bowl.
2. Carefully mix the salad.

per serving: 90 calories, 3.3g protein, 12.8g carbohydrates, 4.4g fat, 3.6g fiber, 0mg cholesterol, 24mg sodium, 721mg potassium

Salmon Salad

Prep time: 10 minutes | **Cook time:** 0 minutes | **Servings:** 4

- 1-pound salmon fillet, boiled
- 1 white onion, diced
- 1 cup lettuce, chopped
- 1 cup spinach, chopped
- 1 tablespoon lemon juice
- 1 teaspoon olive oil
- 1 teaspoon ground paprika

1. Put salmon fillet, onion, lettuce, spinach, and ground paprika, in the salad bowl. Shake the mixture.
2. Then sprinkle the salad with olive oil and lemon juice,.

per serving: 177 calories, 22.7g protein, 3.6g carbohydrates, 8.4g fat, 1.1g fiber, 3.6mg cholesterol, 59mg sodium, 554mg potassium

Yogurt and Radish Salad

Prep time: 10 minutes | **Cook time:** 0 minutes | **Servings:** 4

- 2 cups radishes, sliced
- ½ cup plain yogurt
- 2 tablespoons fresh dill, chopped
- 1 cucumber, chopped
- 1 oz chives, chopped

1. Put all ingredients in the salad bowl.
2. Stir the salad until homogenous.

per serving: 48 calories, 3.2g protein, 8g carbohydrates, 0.6g fat, 1.7g fiber, 2mg cholesterol, 49mg sodium, 390mg potassium

Banana Salad

Prep time: 10 minutes | **Cook time:** 0 minutes | **Servings:** 6

- 5 bananas, chopped
- 2 oranges, peeled, chopped
- 3 tablespoons raw honey
- 1 tablespoon lemon juice

1. Mix bananas with oranges, and lemon juice.
2. Top the salad with raw honey.

per serving: 149 calories, 1.7g protein, 38.4g carbohydrates, 0.4g fat, 4.1g fiber, 0mg cholesterol, 2mg sodium, 472mg potassium

Cucumber Salad

Prep time: 10 minutes | **Cook time:** 0 minutes | **Servings:** 4

- 1 red onion, sliced
- 6 cucumbers, chopped
- 2 tablespoons lemon juice
- 1 tablespoon olive oil
- 1 teaspoon cayenne pepper

1. Mix red onion with cucumber in the salad bowl.
2. Sprinkle the mixture with lemon juice, olive oil, and cayenne pepper.
3. Stir the salad gently.

per serving: 112 calories, 3.3g protein, 19.4g carbohydrates, 4.2g fat, 3g fiber, 0mg cholesterol, 12mg sodium, 722mg potassium

Chives Salad

Prep time: 5 minutes | **Cook time:** 0 minutes | **Servings:** 4

- 4 eggs, boiled, peeled, chopped
- 8 oz chives, chopped
- 1 cucumber, chopped
- ¼ cup coconut cream
- 1 teaspoon ground black pepper

1. Mix chives with eggs, cucumber, and ground black pepper.
2. Add coconut cream.
3. Carefully mix the salad.

per serving: 127 calories, 8.3g protein, 6.7g carbohydrates, 8.5g fat, 2.3g fiber, 164mg cholesterol, 67mg sodium, 384mg potassium

Slaw

Prep time: 10 minutes | **Cook time:** 0 minutes | **Servings:** 4

- 1 carrot, grated
- 2 cups white cabbage, shredded
- 1 apple, chopped
- 1 tablespoon olive oil
- 2 tablespoons lemon juice
- ½ teaspoon ground clove

1. Put all ingredients in the salad bowl and carefully mix.
2. Leave the salad for at least 5 minutes to rest before serving.

per serving: 77 calories, 0.8g protein, 11.6g carbohydrates, 3.8g fat, 2.7g fiber, 0mg cholesterol, 19mg sodium, 180mg potassium

Apple Salad

Prep time: 5 minutes | **Cook time:** 0 minutes | **Servings:** 4

- 2 apples, chopped
- 2 oz raisins, chopped
- 1 tablespoon lemon juice
- 1 tablespoon raw
- honey
- ½ teaspoon ground cinnamon
- 1 carambola, chopped

1. Mix apples with raisins and carambola.
2. Add ground cinnamon, raw honey, and lemon juice.
3. Stir the salad well.

per serving: 128 calories, 1.1g protein, 33.4g carbohydrates, 0.4g fat, 4.3g fiber, 0mg cholesterol, 4mg sodium, 276mg potassium

Spinach Salad

Prep time: 5 minutes | **Cook time:** 0 minutes | **Servings:** 4

- 2 cups spinach, chopped
- 3 tablespoons lemon juice
- 1 cup tomatoes, chopped
- 1 tablespoon olive oil
- ¼ teaspoon ground clove

1. Mix spinach with lemon juice, tomatoes, and olive oil.
2. Top the salad with ground clove and put it in the serving plates.

per serving: 45 calories, 0.9g protein, 2.6g carbohydrates, 3.8g fat, 1g fiber, 0mg cholesterol, 17mg sodium, 206mg potassium

Mint Salad

Prep time: 10 minutes | **Cook time:** 0 minutes | **Servings:** 4

- 1 tablespoon fresh mint, chopped
- 3 oz scallions, chopped
- 3 cups green cabbage, shredded
- 1 tablespoon lemon juice
- 1 tablespoon olive oil
- 1 tablespoon cranberries

1. Put all ingredients in the salad bowl.
2. Gently shake the salad.

per serving: 52 calories, 1.1g protein, 5g carbohydrates, 3.6g fat, 2g fiber, 0mg cholesterol, 14mg sodium, 162mg potassium

Chicken Salad

Prep time: 10 minutes | **Cook time:** 0 minutes | **Servings:** 4

- 1-pound chicken breast, skinless, boneless, boiled
- 2 cups lettuce, chopped
- 2 oz Parmesan, grated
- 2 tablespoons coconut cream
- ½ teaspoon ground black pepper

1. Mix lettuce with chicken breast, coconut cream, and ground black pepper.
2. Top the cooked salad with Parmesan.

per serving: 196 calories, 28.9g protein, 1.9g carbohydrates, 7.7g fat, 0.4g fiber, 83mg cholesterol, 192mg sodium, 481mg potassium

Chives Salad

Prep time: 10 minutes | **Cook time:** 0 minutes | **Servings:** 4

- 6 oz chives, chopped
- 2 tomatoes, chopped
- 1 onion, sliced
- 1 tablespoon olive oil
- 1 tablespoon fresh parsley, chopped

1. Mix chives with tomatoes, parsley, and onion.
2. Then sprinkle the salad with olive oil.
3. Stir it before serving.

per serving: 65 calories, 2.3g protein, 6.9g carbohydrates, 4g fat, 2.4g fiber, 0mg cholesterol, 6mg sodium, 317mg potassium

Fish Salad

Prep time: 10 minutes | **Cook time:** 0 minutes | **Servings:** 4

- 1 pound trout, boiled, chopped
- 1 cup spinach
- 2 tablespoons lime juice
- 2 tomatoes, cubed
- 1 avocado, peeled, pitted and cubed
- 1 tablespoon chives, minced
- 1 tablespoon olive oil

1. Chop the spinach and mix it with trout, lime juice, tomatoes, avocado, and chives.
2. Sprinkle the salad with olive oil.

per serving: 363 calories, 31.9g protein, 7.5g carbohydrates, 23.1g fat, 4.3g fiber, 84mg cholesterol, 89mg sodium, 964mg potassium

Seafood Salad

Prep time: 5 minutes | **Cook time:** 0 minutes | **Servings:** 4

- 3 tablespoons lemon juice
- 2 tablespoons olive oil
- 2 garlic cloves, minced
- 1 pound shrimp, cooked, peeled, boiled
- 5 tomatoes, chopped
- ½ red onion, sliced
- 1 cup lettuce, chopped

1. Put all ingredients in the salad bowl.
2. Carefully mix the salad before serving.

per serving: 235 calories, 27.6g protein, 10.1g carbohydrates, 9.4g fat, 2.3g fiber, 239mg cholesterol, 288mg sodium, 616mg potassium

Watermelon Salad

Prep time: 10 minutes | **Cook time:** 0 minutes | **Servings:** 4

- 3 cups watermelon, chopped
- 2 tablespoons fresh dill, chopped
- ½ teaspoon dried sage
- 2 tablespoons lemon juice
- 1 teaspoon coconut cream
- 1 teaspoon coconut shred

1. Put the watermelon in the salad bowl.
2. Sprinkle it with fresh dill, dried sage, lemon juice, coconut cream, and coconut shred.

per serving: 47 calories, 1.1g protein, 9.9g carbohydrates, 1g fat, 0.8g fiber, 0mg cholesterol, 7mg sodium, 192mg potassium

Crab Salad

Prep time: 5 minutes | **Cook time:** 0 minutes | **Servings:** 4

- 1 cup canned crab meat, drained
- 2 cups arugula, chopped
- 2 oz blackberries
- 1 tablespoon lemon juice
- 1 tablespoon olive oil
- ½ teaspoon lemon zest, grated

1. Mix crab meat with arugula, lemon juice, olive oil, and lemon zest.
2. Top the salad with blackberries.

per serving: 46 calories, 1.4g protein, 2g carbohydrates, 3.8g fat, 1g fiber, 4mg cholesterol, 47mg sodium, 65mg potassium

Seafood and Mango Salad

Prep time: 5 minutes | **Cook time:** 0 minutes | **Servings:** 4

- 1 pound shrimp, cooked, peeled and deveined
- 2 mangoes, peeled and cubed
- 1 tablespoon lemon juice
- 1 teaspoon olive oil
- ½ teaspoon dried rosemary

1. Mix shrimps with mangoes, lemon juice, and olive oil.
2. Top the salad with dried rosemary.

per serving: 247 calories, 27.3g protein, 27.1g carbohydrates, 3.8g fat, 2.8g fiber, 239mg cholesterol, 279mg sodium, 481mg potassium

Arugula and Shrimps Salad

Prep time: 5 minutes | **Cook time:** 0 minutes | **Servings:** 4

- 1 cup shrimp, peeled, deveined and cooked
- 2 cups arugula
- 2 oz Romano cheese, chopped
- 1 tablespoon raw honey
- 1 tablespoon olive oil
- 1 oz pistachios, chopped

1. Mix arugula with shrimps, olive oil, Romano cheese, and pistachios.
2. Sprinkle the salad with raw honey.

per serving: 171 calories, 12.7g protein, 7.1g carbohydrates, 10.9g fat, 0.9g fiber, 137mg cholesterol, 426mg sodium, 125mg potassium

Berries Salad

Prep time: 10 minutes | **Cook time:** 0 minutes | **Servings:** 4

- 1 cup strawberries, chopped
- 1 cup raspberries, chopped
- 1 tablespoon raw honey
- 2 tablespoons coconut cream

1. Mix strawberries with raspberries, and coconut cream.
2. Sprinkle the salad with raw honey.

per serving: 61 calories, 0.8g protein, 11.2g carbohydrates, 2.1g fat, 2.9g fiber, 0mg cholesterol, 2mg sodium, 124mg potassium

Dates Salad

Prep time: 10 minutes | **Cook time:** 0 minutes | **Servings:** 4

- 1 pound shrimp, cooked, peeled and deveined
- 2 cups lettuce, chopped
- 2 tablespoons pistachios, chopped
- 3 tomatoes, chopped
- 1 tablespoon lime juice
- ½ cup dates, chopped
- 2 tablespoons olive oil

1. Put all ingredients in the salad bowl and gently mix.

per serving: 289 calories, 27.8g protein, 23.6g carbohydrates, 10.1g fat, 3.3g fiber, 239mg cholesterol, 294mg sodium, 618mg potassium

Watercress Salad

Prep time: 10 minutes | **Cook time:** 0 minutes | **Servings:** 4

- 1 pound cod fillet, boiled, chopped
- 1 oz chives, chopped
- 2 tablespoons olive oil
- 2 cup watercress
- 1 tablespoon lime juice
- 1 cucumber, chopped
- 1 avocado, peeled, pitted and roughly cubed

1. Mix the ingredients from the list above in the salad bowl.

per serving: 271 calories, 22.4g protein, 1.2g carbohydrates, 7.7g fat, 18g fiber, 56mg cholesterol, 87mg sodium, 410mg potassium

Cantaloupe Salad

Prep time: 5 minutes | **Cook time:** 0 minutes | **Servings:** 2

- 1 cup cantaloupe, peeled and cubed
- 2 oz raisins, chopped
- 2 tablespoons mint, chopped
- 1 tablespoon honey
- 1 teaspoon lime juice

1. Mix all ingredients in the salad bowl.

per serving: 147 calories, 1.8g protein, 38.5g carbohydrates, 0.3g fat, 2.2g fiber, 0mg cholesterol, 19mg sodium, 458mg potassium

Carrot Salad

Prep time: 10 minutes | **Cook time:** 0 minutes | **Servings:** 4

- 3 carrots, spiralized
- ½ cup apricots, pitted, chopped
- 1 tablespoon raw honey
- 2 oz walnuts, chopped
- ½ tablespoon chia seeds

1. Put the carrot in the salad bowl.
2. Add apricots, walnuts, and chia seeds.
3. Shake the salad and top it with raw honey.

per serving: 140 calories, 4.4g protein, 13.1g carbohydrates, 9g fat, 3.1g fiber, 0mg cholesterol, 33mg sodium, 280mg potassium

Eggplant Salad

Prep time: 10 minutes | **Cook time:** 4 minutes | **Servings:** 4

- 3 eggplants, peeled, chopped
- 1 teaspoon salt
- 2 teaspoons minced garlic
- 1 tablespoon olive oil
- 1 tablespoon fresh cilantro, chopped

1. Sprinkle the eggplants with salt and olive oil.
2. Then grill them at 400F for 2 minutes per side.
3. Mix the grilled eggplants with minced garlic and fresh cilantro.

per serving: 135 calories, 4.1g protein, 24.6g carbohydrates, 4.3g fat, 14.6g fiber, 0mg cholesterol, 590mg sodium, 948mg potassium

Avocado Salad

Prep time: 10 minutes | **Cook time:** 0 minutes | **Servings:** 4

- 1 avocado, pitted, peeled, chopped
- 1 teaspoon minced garlic
- 2 tomatoes, chopped
- 1 tablespoon olive oil

1. Put all ingredients in the salad bowl.
2. Carefully mix the salad.

per serving: 145 calories, 1.5g protein, 6.9g carbohydrates, 13.4g fat, 4.1g fiber, 0mg cholesterol, 6mg sodium, 392mg potassium

Quinoa Salad

Prep time: 10 minutes | **Cook time:** 0 minutes | **Servings:** 4

- 1 cup quinoa, cooked
- ¼ cup cranberries
- 1 tablespoon raw honey
- 2 tablespoons lemon juice
- ½ cup grapes, chopped

1. In the salad bowl, mix quinoa with cranberries, raw honey, lemon juice, and grapes.
2. Shake the salad before serving.

per serving: 186 calories, 6.2g protein, 34.4g carbohydrates, 2.g fat, 3.4g fiber, 0mg cholesterol, 4mg sodium, 285mg potassium

Sliced Salad

Prep time: 10 minutes | **Cook time:** 0 minutes | **Servings:** 4

- 2 tomatoes, sliced
- 1 cup parsley, chopped
- 2 avocados, peeled, pitted, sliced
- 2 mangos, peeled, sliced
- 3 tablespoons olive oil

1. Mix tomatoes with parsley in the salad bowl.
2. Add avocados, mangos, and shake the salad.
3. Then sprinkle the salad with olive oil.

per serving: 412 calories, 4.3g protein, 37.2g carbohydrates, 31g fat, 10.7g fiber, 0mg cholesterol, 19mg sodium, 999mg potassium

Turmeric Salad

Prep time: 10 minutes | **Cook time:** 0 minutes | **Servings:** 4

- 2 cups Brussel sprouts, shredded, boiled
- 1 teaspoon ground turmeric
- 1 teaspoon lemon juice
- 1 teaspoon olive oil
- 1 oz almonds, chopped

1. Mix Brussel sprouts with almonds.
2. Then sprinkle the mixture with ground turmeric, lemon juice, and olive oil.
3. Shake the salad well.

per serving: 72 calories, 3.1g protein, 5.9g carbohydrates, 4.9g fat, 2.7g fiber, 0mg cholesterol, 12mg sodium, 238mg potassium

Corn Salad

Prep time: 10 minutes | **Cook time:** 0 minutes | **Servings:** 4

- 1 cup tomatoes, chopped
- 1 cup cucumbers, chopped
- 1 cup corn kernels
- ½ cup green olives,
- chopped
- 1 tablespoon olive oil
- 1 teaspoon minced garlic

1. Put the tomatoes in the salad bowl.
2. Add cucumbers, corn kernels, green olives, and minced garlic.
3. Then sprinkle the salad with olive oil and shake well.

per serving: 122 calories, 6.6g protein, 11g carbohydrates, 6.8g fat, 2.4g fiber, 14mg cholesterol, 81mg sodium, 252mg potassium

Celery Stalk Salad

Prep time: 10 minutes | **Cook time:** 0 minutes | **Servings:** 4

- 16 oz celery stalk, chopped
- 1 orange, peeled, chopped
- 1 red onion, sliced
- 4 oz tofu, cubed
- 2 tablespoons olive oil
- 1 teaspoon lemon juice

1. Put all ingredients in the salad bowl.
2. Shake the salad well.

per serving: 131 calories, 3.8g protein, 11.9g carbohydrates, 8.5g fat, 3.8g fiber, 0mg cholesterol, 95mg sodium, 462mg potassium

Endive Salad

Prep time: 10 minutes | **Cook time:** 0 minutes | **Servings:** 4

- 1 teaspoon onion, diced
- 2 tablespoons lemon juice
- 1 teaspoon coconut cream
- 1 teaspoon raw honey
- 1-pound endives, chopped
- 2 tablespoons olive oil

1. Put all ingredients in the salad bowl.
2. Carefully mix the salad.

per serving: 90 calories, 1.5g protein, 5.6g carbohydrates, 7.6g fat, 3.6g fiber, 0mg cholesterol, 27mg sodium, 371mg potassium

Mushroom Salad

Prep time: 10 minutes | **Cook time:** 0 minutes | **Servings:** 4

- 2 cups mushrooms, sliced, roasted
- 2 onions, sliced, roasted
- 2 eggs, hard-boiled, peeled,
- chopped
- ¼ cup coconut cream
- 1 tablespoon olive oil
- 1 teaspoon ground nutmeg

1. Mix mushrooms with onions in the salad bowl.
2. Add eggs, coconut cream, olive oil, and ground nutmeg.
3. Mix the salad well.

per serving: 128 calories, 4.9g protein, 17.6g carbohydrates, 9.6g fat, 2g fiber, 37mg cholesterol, 37mg sodium, 262mg potassium

Lemon and Radish Salad

Prep time: 10 minutes | **Cook time:** 0 minutes | **Servings:** 4

- 3 cups radish, roughly chopped
- ½ cup fresh cilantro, chopped
- 2 tablespoons
- lemon juice
- 1 tablespoon olive oil
- ½ teaspoon chili powder

1. Put the radish in the salad bowl.
2. Add cilantro, lemon juice, olive oil, and chili powder,
3. Stir the salad well.

per serving: 47 calories, 0.7g protein, 3.4g carbohydrates, 3.7g fat, 1.6g fiber, 0mg cholesterol, 40mg sodium, 229mg potassium

Napa Cabbage Salad

Prep time: 10 minutes | **Cook time:** 0 minutes | **Servings:** 4

- 4 cups napa cabbage, shredded
- 2 oz scallions, chopped
- 2 tablespoons
- lemon juice
- 1 tablespoon olive oil
- ½ teaspoon cayenne pepper

1. Put all ingredients in the salad bowl.
2. Carefully mix the salad.

per serving: 46 calories, 1.4g protein, 2.9g carbohydrates, 3.8g fat, 1.2g fiber, 0mg cholesterol, 49mg sodium, 230mg potassium

Crushed Cucumbers Salad

Prep time: 15 minutes | **Cook time:** 0 minutes | **Servings:** 4

- 5 cucumbers, crushed
- 3 tablespoons lemon juice
- ½ tablespoon olive oil
- 2 garlic cloves, diced
- 1 teaspoon ground clove
- 2 tablespoons dried oregano

1. Put the cucumbers in the salad bowl.
2. Add lemon juice, olive oil, garlic cloves, ground clove, and dried oregano.
3. Shake the salad well and leave it for 10 minutes to marinate.

per serving: 85 calories, 2.9g protein, 16.2g carbohydrates, 2.6g fat, 3.1g fiber, 0mg cholesterol, 12mg sodium, 617mg potassium

Pepper and Corn Salad

Prep time: 10 minutes | **Cook time:** 0 minutes | **Servings:** 4

- 1 cup pepper, chopped
- 1 cup corn kernels, cooked
- 1 teaspoon ground coriander
- 1 tablespoon olive oil

1. Put all ingredients in the salad bowl and carefully mix.

per serving: 88 calories, 2.3g protein, 13.5g carbohydrates, 4.3g fat, 3.6g fiber, 0mg cholesterol, 10mg sodium, 225mg potassium

Almond Salad

Prep time: 10 minutes | **Cook time:** 0 minutes | **Servings:** 4

- 3 cups tomatoes, chopped
- 1 cup cucumbers, chopped
- 2 oz almonds, chopped
- 1 tablespoon olive oil
- 1 tablespoon lemon juice
- 1 teaspoon ground black pepper

1. Mix the tomatoes and cucumbers in the salad bowl.
2. Add almonds, olive oil, lemon juice, and ground black pepper.
3. Shake the salad.

per serving: 142 calories, 4.5g protein, 9.7g carbohydrates, 10.9g fat, 3.7g fiber, 0mg cholesterol, 8mg sodium, 473mg potassium

Zucchini Salad

Prep time: 10 minutes | **Cook time:** 0 minutes | **Servings:** 4

- 4 zucchinis, spiralized
- 2 carrots, spiralized
- 2 tablespoons lemon juice
- 1 tablespoon olive
- oil
- ½ teaspoon ground coriander
- 1 teaspoon ground black pepper
- ¼ teaspoon ground nutmeg

1. Put all ingredients in the salad bowl.
2. Carefully mix the salad.

per serving: 78 calories, 2.8g protein, 10.1g carbohydrates, 4g fat, 3.1g fiber, 0mg cholesterol, 42mg sodium, 628mg potassium

Orange Salad

Prep time: 10 minutes | **Cook time:** 0 minutes | **Servings:** 4

- 3 oranges, peeled, chopped
- 2 kiwis, peeled, chopped
- 2 bananas, peeled, chopped
- 3 tablespoons coconut cream
- 1 tablespoon coconut shred

1. Mix oranges with kiwis and bananas in the salad bowl.
2. Then add coconut cream and coconut shred.

per serving: 179 calories, 2.6g protein, 36.4g carbohydrates, 4.5g fat, 6.5g fiber, 0mg cholesterol, 4mg sodium, 609mg potassium

Snap Pea Salad

Prep time: 10 minutes | **Cook time:** 12 minutes | **Servings:** 4

- 3 cups snap peas, cooked
- 1-pound shrimps, cooked, peeled
- 2 tablespoons olive
- oil
- 1 tablespoon lemon juice
- 1 teaspoon lemon zest, grated

1. Mix snap peas with shrimps in the salad bowl.
2. Add olive oil, lemon juice, and lemon zest.
3. Stir the salad well.

per serving: 284 calories, 31.8g protein, 17.6g carbohydrates, 9.4g fat, 5.6g fiber, 239mg cholesterol, 283mg sodium, 464mg potassium

Noodle Salad

Prep time: 10 minutes | **Cook time:** 0 minutes | **Servings:** 4

- 2 cucumbers, spiralized
- 2 carrots, spiralized
- 1 tablespoon olive oil
- ½ teaspoon ground cumin

1. Mix cucumbers with carrots in the salad bowl.
2. Top the mixture with olive oil and ground cumin.

per serving: 66 calories, 1.3g protein, 8.6g carbohydrates, 3.7g fat, 1.5g fiber, 0mg cholesterol, 24mg sodium, 323mg potassium

Greek Style Salad

Prep time: 20 minutes | **Cook time:** 0 minutes | **Servings:** 4

- 3 cucumbers, chopped
- 3 tomatoes, chopped
- 1 red onion, sliced
- 5 oz tofu, cubed
- 1 tablespoon olive oil
- 1 teaspoon Italian seasonings

1. Put all ingredients in the salad bowl and carefully mix.
2. Leave the salad for 15 minutes in the fridge to marinate.

per serving: 120 calories, 5.5g protein, 15.1g carbohydrates, 5.8g fat, 3.2g fiber, 1mg cholesterol, 15mg sodium, 644mg potassium

Fennel Salad

Prep time: 10 minutes | **Cook time:** 0 minutes | **Servings:** 4

- 12 oz fennel bulb, peeled, chopped
- 1 tablespoon olive oil
- 1 teaspoon lemon juice
- 1 teaspoon ground nutmeg
- 2 oz strawberries, chopped

1. Put the fennel bulb in the salad bowl.
2. Add olive oil, lemon juice, ground nutmeg, and strawberries.
3. Stir the salad well.

per serving: 64 calories, 1.2g protein, 7.6g carbohydrates, 3.9g fat, 3g fiber, 0mg cholesterol, 45mg sodium, 377mg potassium

Oregano Chicken Salad

Prep time: 10 minutes | **Cook time:** 20 minutes | **Servings:** 4

- 12 oz chicken fillet, cooked, chopped
- 1 tablespoon dried oregano
- 1 teaspoon olive oil
- 1 tablespoon lemon juice
- 2 cucumbers, chopped

1. Mix chicken fillet with dried oregano, olive oil, lemon juice, and cucumbers.

per serving: 199 calories, 25.7g protein, 6.3g carbohydrates, 7.8g fat, 1.3g fiber, 76mg cholesterol, 77mg sodium, 451mg potassium

Mustard Salad

Prep time: 10 minutes | **Cook time:** 0 minutes | **Servings:** 2

- 1 teaspoon mustard seeds
- 1 tablespoon mustard
- 1 cup lettuce, chopped
- 1 cup arugula, chopped
- ¼ cup coconut cream
- 1 tablespoon lemon juice
- 1 cucumber, chopped

1. Mix mustard with mustard seeds and put in the salad bowl.
2. Add lettuce, arugula, coconut cream, lemon juice, and cucumber.
3. Shake the salad well.

per serving: 113 calories, 2.9g protein, 9.5g carbohydrates, 8.3g fat, 2.3g fiber, 0mg cholesterol, 102mg sodium, 407mg potassium

Bulgur Salad

Prep time: 10 minutes | **Cook time:** 0 minutes | **Servings:** 4

- 1 cup bulgur, cooked
- 1 chili pepper, chopped
- 1 tablespoon olive oil
- 2 cucumbers, chopped
- ¼ cup coconut cream
- 1 teaspoon ground clove

1. Mix the bulgur with chili pepper in the salad bowl.
2. Add olive oil, cucumbers, coconut cream, and ground clove.
3. Stir the salad well.

per serving: 209 calories, 5.7g protein, 33.3g carbohydrates, 7.8g fat, 7.7g fiber, 0mg cholesterol, 13mg sodium, 412mg potassium

Okra Salad

Prep time: 10 minutes | **Cook time:** 10 minutes | **Servings:** 4

- 1 pound okra, chopped
- 1 cup red kidney beans, cooked
- 3 cucumbers, chopped
- 2 tablespoons olive oil
- 1 tablespoon avocado oil
- 1 tablespoon dried cilantro

1. Put the okra in the saucepan. Add olive oil
2. Roast the okra for 10 minutes on medium heat.
3. Then put the okra in the salad bowl.
4. Add red kidney beans, cucumbers, avocado oil, and dried cilantro.
5. Stir the salad well.

per serving: 299 calories, 14.1g protein, 45g carbohydrates, 8.4g fat, 11.9g fiber, 0mg cholesterol, 18mg sodium, 1308mg potassium

Asparagus Bowl

Prep time: 15 minutes | **Cook time:** 0 minutes | **Servings:** 4

- 1-pound asparagus, chopped, baked
- 6 oz tofu, cubed
- 1 tablespoon chia seeds
- 1 tablespoon olive oil
- 1 tablespoon lemon juice
- 1 oz parsley, chopped

1. Mix tofu with lemon juice and olive oil.
2. Then put the asparagus in the salad bowl
3. Add chia seeds and parsley.
4. After this, add tofu mixture and gently stir the salad.

per serving: 120 calories, 7.4g protein, 8.6g carbohydrates, 7.7g fat, 5.5g fiber, 0mg cholesterol, 13mg sodium, 365mg potassium

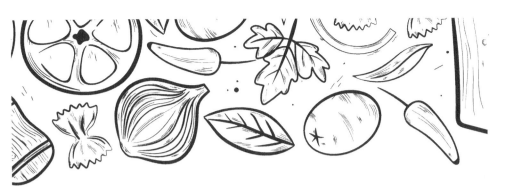

Poultry

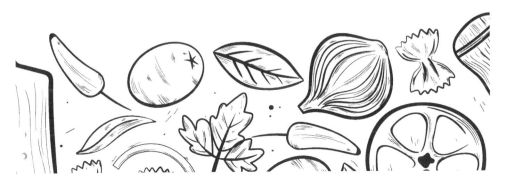

Thyme Chicken

Prep time: 10 minutes | **Cook time:** 35 minutes | **Servings:** 4

- 2-pound chicken wings, boneless
- 1 tablespoon dried thyme
- 2 tablespoons olive oil

1. Mix chicken wings with dried thyme and olive oil and put in the tray.
2. Cook the chicken wings at 365F for 35 minutes.

per serving: 493 calories, 65.7g protein, 0.4g carbohydrates, 23.9g fat, 0.3g fiber, 202mg cholesterol, 195mg sodium, 557mg potassium

Lime Turkey

Prep time: 10 minutes | **Cook time:** 35 minutes | **Servings:** 4

- 1 lime
- 1-pound turkey fillet, chopped
- 1 cup coconut cream
- 1 teaspoon ground nutmeg

1. Chop the lime and put it in the saucepan.
2. Add coconut cream and ground nutmeg.
3. Then add turkey fillet and close the lid.
4. Cook the meal on medium heat for 35 minutes.

per serving: 361 calories, 34.3g protein, 5.4g carbohydrates, 22.9g fat, 1.9g fiber, 101mg cholesterol, 107mg sodium, 452mg potassium

Baked Turkey Fillet

Prep time: 10 minutes | **Cook time:** 35 minutes | **Servings:** 4

- 2 onions, sliced
- 1 tablespoon olive oil
- 1-pound turkey fillet, sliced
- 1 teaspoon dried rosemary
- 1 teaspoon ground black pepper

1. Line the baking tray with baking paper.
2. Then mix turkey fillet with olive oil, onions, dried rosemary, and ground black pepper.
3. Put the mixture in the tray and bake at 360F for 35 minutes.

per serving: 162 calories, 22.2g protein, 7.9g carbohydrates, 4.8g fat, 1.5g fiber, 0mg cholesterol, 3mg sodium, 90mg potassium

Hot Chicken

Prep time: 10 minutes | **Cook time:** 15 minutes | **Servings:** 4

- 2 pounds chicken breast, skinless, boneless and sliced
- 2 chili peppers, chopped
- 1 cup tomatoes, chopped
- 1 tablespoon olive oil

1. Preheat the olive oil in the saucepan.
2. Add chili peppers and tomatoes. Roast them for 5 minutes.
3. Then add chicken breast and carefully mix.
4. Close the lid and cook the chicken on medium heat for 10 minutes.

per serving: 297 calories, 48.5g protein, 1.9g carbohydrates, 9.3g fat, 0.6g fiber, 145mg cholesterol, 118mg sodium, 950mg potassium

Basil Turkey

Prep time: 10 minutes | **Cook time:** 40 minutes | **Servings:** 4

- 2 pounds turkey breast, skinless, boneless and cubed
- 1 tablespoon fresh basil, chopped
- 1 teaspoon ground nutmeg
- 2 tablespoons olive oil

1. Sprinkle the turkey with basil and ground nutmeg.
2. Then sprinkle it with olive oil and put it in the tray.
3. Flatten the turkey pieces well and bake at 355F for 40 minutes.

per serving: 299 calories, 38.8g protein, 9.8g carbohydrates, 11g fat, 1.3g fiber, 98mg cholesterol, 689mg sodium, 2302mg potassium

Fennel Chicken

Prep time: 5 minutes | **Cook time:** 35 minutes | **Servings:** 4

- 2-pounds chicken thighs, skinless
- 8 oz fennel bulb, chopped
- 2 tablespoons olive oil
- 1 teaspoon minced garlic
- 1 tablespoon fennel seeds

1. Mix all ingredients in the mixing bowl.
2. Then transfer the mixture in the lined with the baking paper tray and bake the meal at 365F for 35 minutes.

per serving: 515 calories, 66.6g protein, 5.1g carbohydrates, 24.1g fat, 2.4g fiber, 202mg cholesterol, 226mg sodium, 813mg potassium

Mint Chicken

Prep time: 10 minutes | **Cook time:** 30 minutes | **Servings:** 4

- 2-pound chicken fillet, chopped
- 1 tablespoon mint, chopped
- 1 teaspoon ground
- black pepper
- ½ teaspoon ground turmeric
- ¼ cup of water

1. Mix chicken fillet with mint, ground black pepper, and ground turmeric.
2. Put the chicken in the baking pan, add water, and bake it at 365F for 30 minutes.

per serving: 434 calories, 65.7g protein, 0.6g carbohydrates, 16.9g fat, 0.3g fiber, 202mg cholesterol, 196mg sodium, 572mg potassium

Turkey and Quinoa Bowl

Prep time: 10 minutes | **Cook time:** 30 minutes | **Servings:** 4

- 1-pound turkey breast, skinless, boneless and sliced
- 1 cup quinoa
- 3 cups of water
- 1 teaspoon dried
- rosemary
- ½ teaspoon dried sage
- 1 tablespoon olive oil

1. Mix quinoa with water and cook it for 15 minutes or until the quinoa is soft.
2. Meanwhile, mix turkey with dried rosemary, dried sage, and olive oil.
3. Put the turkey in the tray and bake it for 30 minutes.
4. Serve the quinoa and turkey in one bowl.

per serving: 306 calories, 25.4g protein, 32.3g carbohydrates, 8g fat, 3.7g fiber, 49mg cholesterol, 1159mg sodium, 587mg potassium

Chicken with Cherries

Prep time: 5 minutes | **Cook time:** 30 minutes | **Servings:** 4

- 1-pound chicken breasts, skinless, boneless, sliced
- 1 cup cherries, pitted
- ½ teaspoon
- ground black pepper
- ½ teaspoon dried rosemary
- ¼ cup of water

1. Mix the chicken breast with ground black pepper and dried rosemary.
2. Put it in the baking, add cherries, and water.
3. Bake the meal at 365F for 30 minutes.

per serving: 232 calories, 33.1g protein, 3.8g carbohydrates, 8.4g fat, 0.6g fiber, 101mg cholesterol, 101mg sodium, 208mg potassium

Baked Chicken with Grapes

Prep time: 10 minutes | **Cook time:** 40 minutes | **Servings:** 4

- 1 cup grapes, halved
- 1-pound chicken breast, skinless, boneless, chopped
- ¼ cup of water
- 1 teaspoon ground nutmeg
- 1 tablespoon olive oil

1. Mix chicken breast with ground nutmeg and put in the baking tray.
2. Add water and grapes.
3. Cook the chicken in the preheated to 355F oven for 40 minutes.

per serving: 178 calories, 24.2g protein, 4.2g carbohydrates, 6.6g fat, 0.3g fiber, 73mg cholesterol, 59mg sodium, 466mg potassium

Chicken with Asparagus

Prep time: 10 minutes | **Cook time:** 30 minutes | **Servings:** 4

- 1-pound chicken breast, skinless, boneless, chopped
- 10 oz asparagus, chopped
- ½ cup of water
- 1 teaspoon ground ginger
- 1 teaspoon olive oil

1. Pour the olive oil in the saucepan.
2. Mix ground ginger with chicken and put in the oil. Roast it for 3 minutes per side.
3. Then add asparagus and water.
4. Close the lid and cook the meal on medium heat for 25 minutes more.

per serving: 155 calories, 25.6g protein, 3.1g carbohydrates, 4.1g fat, 1.6g fiber, 73mg cholesterol, 60mg sodium, 569mg potassium

Sweet Chicken Bake

Prep time: 10 minutes | **Cook time:** 30 minutes | **Servings:** 4

- 1-pound chicken fillet, chopped
- 1 cup peaches, chopped
- ½ cup of water
- 1 teaspoon ground nutmeg
- 1 teaspoon ground clove
- ½ lemon, chopped

1. Mix the chicken fillet with ground nutmeg and ground clove.
2. Put the chicken in the baking pan.
3. Add water, lemon, and peaches.
4. Close the lid and cook the meal in the oven at 365F for 30 minutes.

per serving: 237 calories, 33.3g protein, 4.8g carbohydrates, 8.8g fat, 1.1g fiber, 101mg cholesterol, 100mg sodium, 365mg potassium

Tomato Chicken

Prep time: 10 minutes | **Cook time:** 25 minutes | **Servings:** 4

- 1 onion, diced
- 2 cups tomatoes, chopped
- 1 chili pepper, chopped
- 1 garlic clove, chopped
- 1 tablespoon olive oil
- 1-pound chicken fillet, chopped

1. Put all ingredients in the saucepan and carefully mix.
2. Close the lid and cook the chicken for 25 minutes on medium heat. Stir the chicken from time to time to avoid burning.

per serving: 274 calories, 34g protein, 6.4g carbohydrates, 12.1g fat, 1.7g fiber, 101mg cholesterol, 103mg sodium, 534mg potassium

Pistachio Chicken

Prep time: 10 minutes | **Cook time:** 45 minutes | **Servings:** 4

- 1 teaspoon garlic, minced
- 2 tablespoons olive oil
- 1-pound chicken thighs, skinless,
- boneless
- 2 oz pistachios, chopped
- 1 teaspoon dried rosemary
- ¼ cup of water

1. Mix chicken thighs with garlic, olive oil, dried rosemary, and pistachios.
2. Put the chicken thighs in the baking pan, add water, and cook them for 45 minutes at 355F.

per serving: 353 calories, 35.7g protein, 4.2g carbohydrates, 22.1g fat, 1.6g fiber, 101mg cholesterol, 174mg sodium, 428mg potassium

Chicken and Beans

Prep time: 5 minutes | **Cook time:** 30 minutes | **Servings:** 4

- 1 cup red kidney beans, cooked
- 1-pound chicken fillet, chopped
- 1 cup of water
- 1 cup tomatoes, chopped
- 1 teaspoon chili powder

1. Put the chicken fillet in the saucepan.
2. Add red kidney beans, water, tomatoes, and chili powder.
3. Close the lid and cook the meal on medium heat for 30 minutes.

per serving: 381 calories, 43.7g protein, 30.3g carbohydrates, 9.1g fat, 7.8g fiber, 101mg cholesterol, 114mg sodium, 1020mg potassium

Chicken with Peppers

Prep time: 10 minutes | **Cook time:** 26 minutes | **Servings:** 4

- 1-pound chicken breast, skinless, boneless, chopped
- 1 cup bell pepper, chopped
- 1 tablespoon olive oil
- 1 teaspoon ground paprika
- ½ cup of water

1. Roast the chicken breast in the olive oil for 3 minutes per side.
2. Add bell peppers, ground paprika, and water.
3. Close the lid and simmer the meal for 20 minutes.

per serving: 170 calories, 24.4g protein, 2.6g carbohydrates, 6.5g fat, 0.6g fiber, 73mg cholesterol, 60mg sodium, 488mg potassium

Chicken with Green Beans

Prep time: 10 minutes | **Cook time:** 40 minutes | **Servings:** 4

- 12 oz green beans, chopped
- 1-pound chicken thighs, skinless, boneless, chopped
- 1 teaspoon chili

- powder
- 2 tablespoons lemon juice
- 2 tablespoons olive oil
- ¼ cup of water

1. Mix chicken thighs with chili powder, lemon juice, and olive oil.
2. Preheat the saucepan and put the chicken inside. Roast it for 5 minutes per side.
3. Then add water and green beans.
4. Close the lid and cook the meal on medium heat for 30 minutes.

per serving: 306 calories, 34.5g protein, 6.6g carbohydrates, 15.7g fat, 3.1g fiber, 101mg cholesterol, 111mg sodium, 475mg potassium

Turmeric Chicken Wings

Prep time: 10 minutes | **Cook time:** 35 minutes | **Servings:** 4

- 8 chicken wings
- 1 tablespoon ground turmeric
- 1 teaspoon minced

- garlic
- 2 tablespoons olive oil
- 1 tomato, crushed

1. Mix chicken wings with ground turmeric, minced garlic, and olive oil.
2. Put the chicken wings in the baking tray, add tomato, and bake the meal at 365F for 35 minutes.

per serving: 267 calories, 18.6g protein, 1.9g carbohydrates, 20.4g fat, 0.6g fiber, 57mg cholesterol, 57mg sodium, 208mg potassium

Baked Chicken Breast

Prep time: 10 minutes | **Cook time:** 40 minutes | **Servings:** 4

- 2-pound chicken breast, skinless, boneless
- 1 tablespoon Italian seasonings
- 2 tablespoons

- lemon juice
- 2 tablespoons olive oil
- ½ teaspoon minced garlic

1. 1. Mix chicken breast with Italian seasonings, lemon juice, olive oil, and minced garlic.
2. Wrap the chicken breast in the foil and bake at 365f for 40 minutes.

per serving: 332 calories, 48.2g protein, 0.7g carbohydrates, 13.8g fat, 0g fiber, 148mg cholesterol, 118mg sodium, 852mg potassium

Tarragon Chicken

Prep time: 10 minutes | **Cook time:** 40 minutes | **Servings:** 4

- 2 tablespoons olive oil
- ½ teaspoon minced garlic
- 1 teaspoon lemon zest, grated

- 1 teaspoon dried tarragon
- 1-pound chicken breast, boneless, skinless

1. Rub the chicken breast with minced garlic, lemon zest, dried tarragon, and olive oil.
2. Put the chicken in the tray and bake it at 360F for 40 minutes.

per serving: 191 calories, 24.1g protein, 0.3g carbohydrates, 9.9g fat, 0.1g fiber, 73mg cholesterol, 58mg sodium, 427mg potassium

Clove Chicken Thighs

Prep time: 10 minutes | **Cook time:** 45 minutes | **Servings:** 4

- 1-pound chicken thighs, skinless, boneless
- 1 tablespoon ground clove

- 1 tablespoon lemon juice
- 1 tablespoon olive oil

1. Mix chicken thighs with ground clove, lemon juice, and olive oil.
2. Put the chicken thighs in the baking tray and bake at 350F for 45 minutes.

per serving: 252 calories, 32.9g protein, 1.1g carbohydrates, 12.3g fat, 0.4g fiber, 0.6mg cholesterol, 102mg sodium, 298mg potassium

Baked Turkey with Apples

Prep time: 10 minutes | **Cook time:** 45 minutes | **Servings:** 4

- 2-pound turkey fillet, chopped
- 1 cup apples, chopped
- 1 teaspoon clove
- 2 garlic cloves, peeled
- 1 cup of water
- 1 tablespoon olive oil

1. Put all ingredients in the saucepan and gently mix.
2. Close the lid and cook the meal on medium heat for 45 minutes.

per serving: 299 calories, 39g protein, 18.1g carbohydrates, 7.5g fat, 2.7g fiber, 98mg cholesterol, 2306mg sodium, 757mg potassium

Chicken and Beets

Prep time: 10 minutes | **Cook time:** 40 minutes | **Servings:** 4

- 10 oz beets, peeled, chopped
- 1-pound chicken breast, skinless, boneless, chopped
- 1 cup of water
- 1 teaspoon dried rosemary
- 1 tablespoon olive oil
- 1 teaspoon ground clove

1. Roast the chicken breast with oil for 5 minutes per side.
2. Then put the chicken in the saucepan.
3. Add beets, water, dried rosemary, and ground clove.
4. Close the lid and cook the meal for 30 minutes.

per serving: 193 calories, 25.3g protein, 7.6g carbohydrates, 6.6g fat, 1.7g fiber, 7.3mg cholesterol, 116mg sodium, 645mg potassium

Spinach Chicken

Prep time: 10 minutes | **Cook time:** 40 minutes | **Servings:** 4

- 1-pound chicken breast, skinless, boneless, chopped
- 2 cups spinach, chopped
- 1 teaspoon minced
- ginger
- 1 teaspoon chili pepper
- 1 cup of coconut milk

1. Put all ingredients in the saucepan and carefully mix.
2. Close the lid and simmer the meal on medium-low heat for 40 minutes.
3. Serve the cooked meal in the bowls.

per serving: 273 calories, 25.9g protein, 4.3g carbohydrates, 17.2g fat, 1.8g fiber, 73mg cholesterol, 79mg sodium, 671mg potassium

Chicken with Strawberries

Prep time: 10 minutes | **Cook time:** 35 minutes | **Servings:** 4

- 1-pound chicken breast, skinless, boneless, chopped
- 1 cup strawberries, chopped
- 1 cup of water
- 1 teaspoon dried mint
- 1 teaspoon chili powder
- 1 tablespoon olive oil

1. Roast the chicken breast with olive oil for 2 minutes per side.
2. Then add strawberries, water, dried mint, and chili powder.
3. Close the lid and cook the meal on medium heat for 30 minutes.

per serving: 173 calories, 24.4g protein, 3.2g carbohydrates, 6.6g fat, 1g fiber, 73mg cholesterol, 67mg sodium, 490mg potassium

Curry Chicken

Prep time: 10 minutes | **Cook time:** 26 minutes | **Servings:** 4

- 1-pound chicken breast, skinless, boneless, chopped
- 1 tablespoon curry paste
- ½ cup of coconut
- milk
- 1 teaspoon lemongrass, chopped
- 1 teaspoon olive oil

1. Mix the curry paste with coconut milk and lemongrass.
2. Roast the chicken with olive oil for 3 minutes per side.
3. Then add coconut milk mixture and stir the meal.
4. Close the lid and cook the chicken on medium heat for 20 minutes.

per serving: 234 calories, 24.9g protein, 2.8g carbohydrates, 13.4g fat, 0.7g fiber, 73mg cholesterol, 62mg sodium, 501mg potassium

Taco Chicken

Prep time: 10 minutes | **Cook time:** 35 minutes | **Servings:** 4

- 1 tablespoon taco seasonings
- 1-pound chicken breast, skinless, boneless, chopped
- 2 tablespoons olive oil
- 1 tablespoon lemon juice

1. Mix chicken breast with taco seasonings, olive oil, and lemon juice.
2. Put the chicken in the baking tray and flatten well.
3. Bake the chicken at 360F for 35 minutes.

per serving: 195 calories, 24.1g protein, 1.1g carbohydrates, 9.9g fat, 0g fiber, 73mg cholesterol, 164mg sodium, 424mg potassium

Ginger Chicken

Prep time: 5 minutes | **Cook time:** 35 minutes | **Servings:** 4

- 1-pound chicken breast, skinless, boneless, chopped
- 1 tablespoon minced ginger
- 1 teaspoon minced garlic
- ½ cup of water
- 1 teaspoon cayenne pepper

1. Mix chicken breast with minced ginger, minced garlic, and cayenne pepper.
2. Put the chicken in the saucepan. Add water.
3. Cook the chicken on medium heat for 35 minutes.

per serving: 136 calories, 24.3g protein, 1.4g carbohydrates, 3g fat, 0.3g fiber, 73mg cholesterol, 59mg sodium, 450mg potassium

Chili Chicken

Prep time: 10 minutes | **Cook time:** 40 minutes | **Servings:** 4

- 1-pound chicken fillet, sliced
- 1 teaspoon chili flakes
- ½ cup tomatoes, chopped
- ½ cup of water

1. Put all ingredients in the saucepan and close the lid.
2. Cook the chicken on medium heat for 40 minutes.

per serving: 220 calories, 33g protein, 0.9g carbohydrates, 8.5g fat, 0.3g fiber, 101mg cholesterol, 100mg sodium, 330mg potassium

Cinnamon Chicken

Prep time: 10 minutes | **Cook time:** 40 minutes | **Servings:** 4

- 8 chicken wings, skinless, boneless
- 1 teaspoon ground cinnamon
- 2 tablespoons lemon juice
- 1 tablespoon olive oil
- ½ teaspoon lemon zest, grated

1. Mix chicken wings with ground cinnamon, lemon juice, olive oil, and lemon zest.
2. Put the chicken in the tray and bake at 355F for 40 minutes.

per serving: 172 calories, 21.2g protein, 0.7g carbohydrates, 9g fat, 0.4g fiber, 65mg cholesterol, 64mg sodium, 190mg potassium

Lemon Turkey

Prep time: 10 minutes | **Cook time:** 30 minutes | **Servings:** 4

- 1-pound turkey fillet, chopped
- 1 lemon
- 1 teaspoon cayenne pepper
- 1 tablespoon olive oil

1. Mix the turkey fillet with cayenne pepper and olive oil.
2. Then squeeze the lemon in the turkey and transfer the meal in the baking tray.
3. Bake the turkey at 360F for 30 minutes/

per serving: 154 calories, 24g protein, 4.1g carbohydrates, 4.9g fat, 0.5g fiber, 0mg cholesterol, 0mg sodium, 29mg potassium

Honey Chicken Wings

Prep time: 10 minutes | **Cook time:** 1 hour | **Servings:** 4

- 2 pounds' chicken wings, halved
- 2 tablespoons raw honey
- 1 teaspoon chili powder
- 1 tablespoon lemon juice

1. Mix chicken wings with raw honey, chili powder, and lemon juice.
2. Wrap the chicken wings in the foil and put it in the tray.
3. Bake the chicken wings at 350F for 1 hour.

per serving: 466 calories, 65.8g protein, 9.1g carbohydrates, 17g fat, 0.3g fiber, 202mg cholesterol, 203mg sodium, 574mg potassium

Cilantro Chicken

Prep time: 10 minutes | **Cook time:** 20 minutes | **Servings:** 4

- 8 chicken thighs, boneless
- 1 tablespoon dried cilantro
- 1 teaspoon chili powder
- 1 tablespoon olive oil

1. Roast the chicken thighs in the olive oil for 5 minutes per side.
2. Add dried cilantro and chili powder.
3. Close the lid and cook the chicken for 10 minutes more.

per serving: 587 calories, 84.6g protein, 0.4g carbohydrates, 25.3g fat, 0.2g fiber, 260mg cholesterol, 258mg sodium, 723mg potassium

Yogurt Chicken

Prep time: 10 minutes | **Cook time:** 30 minutes | **Servings:** 4

- 1 cup plain yogurt
- 1-pound chicken fillet, chopped
- 1 tablespoon Italian seasonings

1. Mix chicken with Italian seasonings and plain yogurt.
2. Put the chicken in the baking pan and bake at 360F for 30 minutes.

per serving: 270 calories, 36.3g protein, 4.7g carbohydrates, 10.2g fat, 0g fiber, 107mg cholesterol, 142mg sodium, 421mg potassium

Chicken with Zucchinis

Prep time: 10 minutes | **Cook time:** 40 minutes | **Servings:** 4

- 1-pound chicken breast, skinless, boneless, chopped
- 2 zucchinis, chopped
- ½ cup of coconut milk
- ¼ cup of water
- 1 teaspoon ground nutmeg
- 1 teaspoon ground clove

1. Put all ingredients in the casserole mold and gently stir.
2. Place the casserole mold in the oven and cook the meal for 40 minutes at 360F.

per serving: 219 calories, 26g protein, 5.5g carbohydrates, 10.5 fat, 2g fiber, 73mg cholesterol, 74mg sodium, 763mg potassium

Parsley Chicken

Prep time: 10 minutes | **Cook time:** 30 minutes | **Servings:** 4

- 1-pound chicken breast, skinless, boneless, chopped
- 1 cup parsley, chopped
- 1 cup of water
- 1 teaspoon peppercorns

1. Pour water in the saucepan.
2. Add parsley and peppercorns.
3. Then add chicken breast and cook it for 30 minutes on medium heat.

per serving: 136 calories, 24.6g protein, 1.3g carbohydrates, 3g fat, 0.6g fiber, 73mg cholesterol, 68mg sodium, 510mg potassium

Coconut Chicken Wings

Prep time: 10 minutes | **Cook time:** 45 minutes | **Servings:** 4

- 8 chicken wings
- 1 cup coconut cream
- 1 tablespoon coconut shred
- 2 garlic cloves, peeled
- 1 teaspoon dried mint

1. Mix chicken wings with coconut shred, garlic cloves, and dried mint.
2. Put the chicken wings in the saucepan.
3. Add coconut cream and cook the meal on medium-low heat for 45 minutes.

per serving: 350 calories, 19.8g protein, 4.4g carbohydrates, 28.8g fat, 1.6g fiber, 57mg cholesterol, 66mg sodium, 291mg potassium

Corn and Chicken Stew

Prep time: 10 minutes | **Cook time:** 35 minutes | **Servings:** 6

- 2-pound chicken fillet, chopped
- 1 cup corn kernels
- 1 cup of water
- 1 teaspoon peppercorns
- 1 onion, sliced
- 1 teaspoon chili pepper

1. Put all ingredients in the saucepan and stir gently.
2. Close the lid and cook the stew on medium heat for 35 minutes.

per serving: 318 calories, 44.8g protein, 6.9g carbohydrates, 11.5g fat, 1.2g fiber, 135mg cholesterol, 136mg sodium, 471mg potassium

Chicken and Cabbage Bowl

Prep time: 10 minutes | **Cook time:** 40 minutes | **Servings:** 4

- 1 cup white cabbage, shredded
- 1 cup ground chicken
- 1 teaspoon ground black pepper
- 1 teaspoon chili powder
- 1 cup tomatoes, chopped
- ½ cup of water

1. Put all ingredients in the casserole mold and carefully mix.
2. Cook the meal at 360F for 40 minutes.

per serving: 82 calories, 10.9g protein, 3.5g carbohydrates, 2.8g fat, 1.3g fiber, 31mg cholesterol, 43mg sodium, 241mg potassium

Paprika Chicken

Prep time: 10 minutes | **Cook time:** 25 minutes | **Servings:** 4

- 2 tablespoons ground paprika
- 1-pound chicken fillet, sliced
- 2 tablespoons olive oil
- 1 tablespoon apple cider vinegar

1. Mix chicken fillet with ground paprika, olive oil, and apple cider vinegar.
2. Put the chicken in the baking tray and bake at 360F for 25 minutes.

per serving: 286 calories, 33.3g protein, 2g carbohydrates, 15.9g fat, 1.3g fiber, 101mg cholesterol, 99mg sodium, 359mg potassium

Cumin Chicken

Prep time: 10 minutes | **Cook time:** 20 minutes | **Servings:** 4

- 1 tablespoon cumin seeds
- 2 tablespoons olive oil
- 1 teaspoon minced
- garlic
- 1-pound chicken breast, skinless, boneless, chopped
- ¼ cup of water

1. Mix chicken breast with cumin seeds, olive oil, and minced garlic.
2. Put the chicken in the saucepan and roast it for 5 minutes per side.
3. Add water and stir well.
4. Cook the chicken for 10 minutes more.

per serving: 196 calories, 24.4g protein, 0.9g carbohydrates, 10.2g fat, 0.2g fiber, 73mg cholesterol, 61mg sodium, 449mg potassium

Wrapped Chicken

Prep time: 10 minutes | **Cook time:** 20 minutes | **Servings:** 4

- 2 cups ground chicken
- 1 teaspoon ground black pepper
- 1 teaspoon dried
- oregano
- 8 oz kale leaves
- ½ cup of water
- 1 tablespoon olive oil

1. Pour olive oil in the skillet.
2. Add dried oregano, ground black pepper, and ground chicken.
3. Cook the mixture for 10 minutes.
4. Then put the chicken mixture on the kale leaves and wrap them.
5. Put the wrapped kale in the skillet, add water.
6. Close the lid and cook the meal on medium heat for 10 minutes.

per serving: 193 calories, 22g protein, 6.5g carbohydrates, 8.8g fat, 1.2g fiber, 62mg cholesterol, 86mg sodium, 462mg potassium

Orange Chicken

Prep time: 10 minutes | **Cook time:** 25 minutes | **Servings:** 4

- 1-pound chicken fillet, sliced
- 2 oranges, sliced
- 1 tablespoon olive
- oil
- ½ teaspoon dried thyme

1. Mix chicken fillet with olive oil and dried thyme.
2. Put the chicken in the tray in one layer.
3. Top it with sliced oranges and bake at 365F for 25 minutes.

per serving: 289 calories, 33.7g protein, 10.9g carbohydrates, 12g fat, 2.3g fiber, 101mg cholesterol, 98mg sodium, 443mg potassium

Onion Chicken

Prep time: 10 minutes | **Cook time:** 40 minutes | **Servings:** 4

- 1-pound chicken breast, skinless, boneless, chopped
- 1 cup onion, diced
- 2 tablespoons olive oil
- ½ cup of water
- 1 teaspoon cayenne pepper

1. Roast the chicken breast in the olive oil for 2 minutes per side.
2. Then add onion, water, and cayenne pepper.
3. Close the lid and cook the meal on medium-low heat for 40 minutes.

per serving: 202 calories, 24.4g protein, 2.9g carbohydrates, 10g fat, 0.7g fiber, 73mg cholesterol, 60mg sodium, 471mg potassium

Jalapeno Chicken

Prep time: 10 minutes | **Cook time:** 35 minutes | **Servings:** 4

- 3 jalapenos, chopped
- 1-pound chicken breast, skinless, boneless, chopped
- ½ cup of water
- 1 tablespoon minced garlic
- 1 tablespoon dried oregano
- 1 tablespoon olive oil

1. Mix chicken with minced garlic, dried oregano, and olive oil.
2. Put in the saucepan and add jalapenos and water.
3. Close the lid and cook the chicken on medium heat for 35 minutes.

per serving: 169 calories, 29.4g protein, 2g carbohydrates, 6.5g fat, 0.8g fiber, 73mg cholesterol, 59mg sodium, 470mg potassium

Masala Chicken Wings

Prep time: 10 minutes | **Cook time:** 25 minutes | **Servings:** 4

- 1-pound chicken wings, boneless
- 1 tablespoon
- garam masala
- ½ cup coconut cream

1. Pour the coconut cream in the saucepan.
2. Rub the chicken wings with garam masala and put in the coconut cream.
3. Close the lid and cook the meal on medium heat for 25 minutes.

per serving: 284 calories, 33.5g protein, 1.7g carbohydrates, 15.6g fat, 0.7g fiber, 101mg cholesterol, 105mg sodium, 354mg potassium

Chicken Alfredo

Prep time: 10 minutes | **Cook time:** 30 minutes | **Servings:** 4

- 4 oz Alfredo sauce
- ½ cup of water
- 1 carrot, chopped
- 1-pound chicken breast, skinless, boneless, chopped
- 1 teaspoon peppercorns

1. Pour water in the saucepan.
2. Add carrot, chicken breast, and peppercorns.
3. Cook the meal on medium heat for 30 minutes.
4. Then remove the chicken from the water and put in the serving plates.
5. Top the chicken with Alfredo sauce.

per serving: 254 calories, 28.4g protein, 15.3g carbohydrates, 8g fat, 0.5g fiber, 83mg cholesterol, 1450mg sodium, 475mg potassium

Ground Chicken Mix

Prep time: 10 minutes | **Cook time:** 30 minutes | **Servings:** 4

- 2 cups ground chicken
- 2 tablespoons olive oil
- 2 jalapenos, chopped
- 1 teaspoon smoked paprika

1. Put all ingredients in the skillet and carefully mix.
2. Cook the ground chicken mix for 30 minutes on low heat. Stir it from time to time.

per serving: 197 calories, 20.4g protein, 0.7g carbohydrates, 12.3g fat, 0.4g fiber, 6.2mg cholesterol, 60mg sodium, 198mg potassium

Honey Duck Fillet

Prep time: 10 minutes | **Cook time:** 15 minutes | **Servings:** 4

- 1-pound duck fillet, chopped
- 1 tablespoon raw honey
- 1 teaspoon ground turmeric
- ½ teaspoon dried mint
- 1 tablespoon olive oil

1. Mix duck fillet with dried mint and ground turmeric.
2. Then preheat the olive oil and put the duck pieces inside.
3. Roast them for 10 minutes. Stir the meat from time to time.
4. After this, add honey and carefully mix the meal.
5. Close the lid and cook it for 5 minutes more.

per serving: 189 calories, 33.5g protein, 4.7g carbohydrates, 4.2g fat, 0.2g fiber, 0mg cholesterol, 171mg sodium, 89mg potassium

Chicken with Mushrooms

Prep time: 5 minutes | **Cook time:** 45 minutes | **Servings:** 4

- 1-pound chicken breast, skinless, boneless, chopped
- 2 cups mushrooms, chopped
- 1 onion, sliced
- 1 tablespoon olive oil
- ½ cup coconut cream
- 1 cup of water
- 1 teaspoon dried rosemary

1. Pour olive oil in the saucepan.
2. Add mushrooms, dried rosemary, and onion. Roast the ingredients for 3 minutes per side.
3. Then add coconut cream and chopped chicken.
4. Stir the mixture and close the lid.
5. Cook it on medium heat for 40 minutes.

per serving: 248 calories, 26.1g protein, 5.6g carbohydrates, 13.7g fat, 1.7g fiber, 7.3mg cholesterol, 67mg sodium, 653mg potassium

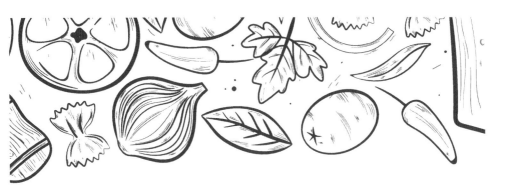

Fish & Seafood

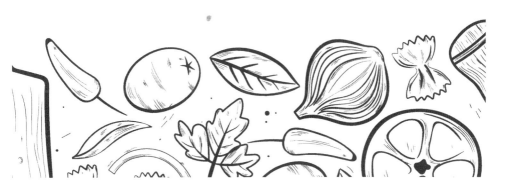

Lemon Flounder

Prep time: 10 minutes | **Cook time:** 35 minutes | **Servings:** 4

- 1-pound flounder
- 1 lemon, sliced
- 2 oz Parmesan, grated
- 1 tablespoon olive oil
- 1 teaspoon dried thyme

1. Mix flounder with dried thyme and olive oil.
2. Put the fish in the foil.
3. Add lemon and Parmesan. Wrap the fish.
4. Bake the flounder at 365F for 35 minutes.

per serving: 213 calories, 32.1g protein, 2g carbohydrates, 8.3g fat, 0.5g fiber, 87mg cholesterol, 251mg sodium, 412mg potassium

Clove Salmon

Prep time: 10 minutes | **Cook time:** 6 minutes | **Servings:** 2

- 10 oz salmon fillet
- 1 teaspoon ground clove
- 1 teaspoon onion powder
- 2 tablespoons olive oil

1. Rub the salmon fillet with ground clove and onion powder.
2. Preheat the olive oil well.
3. Put the salmon in the oil and roast it for 3 minutes per side.

per serving: 315 calories, 27.7g protein, 1.6g carbohydrates, 2.3g fat, 0.4g fiber, 63mg cholesterol, 66mg sodium, 567mg potassium

Date Salmon

Prep time: 10 minutes | **Cook time:** 25 minutes | **Servings:** 4

- 1-pound salmon fillet, chopped
- 4 dates, pitted, chopped
- ½ cup coconut cream
- 1 teaspoon chili flakes

1. Mix salmon with dates, coconut cream, and chili flakes.
2. Put the mixture in the baking pan and bake at 365F for 25 minutes.

per serving: 243 calories, 22.9g protein, 7.9g carbohydrates, 14.2g fat, 1.3g fiber, 50mg cholesterol, 55mg sodium, 570mg potassium

Mango Shrimps

Prep time: 10 minutes | **Cook time:** 15 minutes | **Servings:** 4

- 1-pound shrimps, peeled
- 1 mango, pitted, peeled
- 1 tablespoon olive
- oil
- 1 teaspoon chili powder
- ¼ cup of water

1. Put all ingredients in the saucepan and bring to boil.
2. Simmer the meal for 10 minutes.

per serving: 217 calories, 26.6g protein, 14.7g carbohydrates, 5.9g fat, 1.6g fiber, 239mg cholesterol, 285mg sodium, 346mg potassium

Taco Cod

Prep time: 10 minutes | **Cook time:** 10 minutes | **Servings:** 4

- 1-pound cod fillet, chopped
- 1 tablespoon olive
- oil
- 1 teaspoon taco seasonings

1. Preheat the olive oil well.
2. Mix cod with taco dressing and put in the hot oil.
3. Roast the fish for 10 minutes on medium heat. Stir it from time to time.

per serving: 126 calories, 20.3g protein, 1g carbohydrates, 4.5g fat, 0g fiber, 56mg cholesterol, 176mg sodium, 0mg potassium

Wrap Salmon

Prep time: 10 minutes | **Cook time:** 0 minutes | **Servings:** 4

- 1-pound salmon fillet, boiled
- 4 wonton wraps
- 1 teaspoon chives, chopped
- 1 tablespoon plain yogurt
- ½ teaspoon chili flakes

1. Mix salmon with chives, plain yogurt, and chili flakes.
2. Put the mixture on the wonton wraps and wrap them.

per serving: 163 calories, 22.7g protein, 2.3g carbohydrates, 7.1g fat, 0g fiber, 50mg cholesterol, 53mg sodium, 446mg potassium

Yogurt Shrimp

Prep time: 10 minutes | **Cook time:** 10 minutes | **Servings:** 4

- 1-pound shrimps, peeled
- 1 cup plain yogurt
- 1 teaspoon dried thyme
- 1 teaspoon dried rosemary
- 1 teaspoon olive oil

1. Mix shrimps with plain yogurt, dried thyme, and rosemary.
2. Preheat the olive oil well.
3. Put the shrimp mixture in the oil and roast it for 4 minutes per side.

per serving: 190 calories, 29.4g protein, 6.4g carbohydrates, 3.9g fat, 0.2g fiber, 242mg cholesterol, 320mg sodium, 340mg potassium

Salmon Steaks

Prep time: 10 minutes | **Cook time:** 10 minutes | **Servings:** 2

- 2 salmon steaks
- 1 teaspoon ground black pepper
- 1 tablespoon plain yogurt
- 1 tablespoon olive oil

1. Preheat the grill to 400F.
2. Mix salmon steaks with ground black pepper, plain yogurt, and olive oil.
3. Put the steaks in the hot grill and cook them for 4 minutes per side.

per serving: 304 calories, 35.1g protein, 1.2g carbohydrates, 18.1g fat, 0.3g fiber, 79mg cholesterol, 84mg sodium, 715mg potassium

Mustard Salmon

Prep time: 10 minutes | **Cook time:** 8 minutes | **Servings:** 2

- 12 oz salmon fillet
- 2 tablespoons plain yogurt
- 1 tablespoon mustard
- 1 tablespoon olive oil

1. Mix salmon with mustard and plain yogurt.
2. Then preheat the olive oil well.
3. Put the salmon in hot oil and roast it for 4 minutes per side.

per serving: 322 calories, 35.3g protein, 3g carbohydrates, 19.3g fat, 0.8g fiber, 76mg cholesterol, 86mg sodium, 727mg potassium

Mint Scallops

Prep time: 10 minutes | **Cook time:** 6 minutes | **Servings:** 4

- 1 tablespoon olive oil
- 1 tablespoon fresh mint, blended
- 1-pound scallops
- 1 tablespoon apple cider vinegar

1. Mix scallops with apple cider vinegar and mint.
2. The preheat the olive oil well.
3. Put the scallops in the hot oil and cook them for 3 minutes per side.

per serving: 131 calories, 19.1g protein, 2.g carbohydrates, 4.4g fat, 0.1g fiber, 37mg cholesterol, 183mg sodium, 374mg potassium

Peppercorn Cod

Prep time: 10 minutes | **Cook time:** 10 minutes | **Servings:** 2

- 10 oz cod fillet
- 1 cup of water
- 1 bay leaf
- 1 tablespoon peppercorns

1. Bring the water to boil.
2. Add bay leaf and peppercorns.
3. Then add cod fillet and coil it for 7 minutes.
4. Remove the cooked fillet from the water.

per serving: 123 calories, 25.7g protein, 2.3g carbohydrates, 1.4g fat, 0.9g fiber, 70mg cholesterol, 94mg sodium, 43mg potassium

Honey Salmon

Prep time: 10 minutes | **Cook time:** 20 minutes | **Servings:** 4

- 1-pound salmon fillet, chopped
- 1 teaspoon dried mint
- 1 tablespoon raw honey
- ¼ cup coconut cream
- 1 teaspoon olive oil

1. Mix salmon fillet with dried mint and coconut cream.
2. Pour olive oil in the saucepan.
3. Add salmon and raw honey.
4. Close the lid and cook the fish for 20 minutes.

per serving: 211 calories, 22.4g protein, 5.2g carbohydrates, 11.8g fat, 0.4g fiber, 50mg cholesterol, 53mg sodium, 480mg potassium

Parmesan Tilapia

Prep time: 10 minutes | **Cook time:** 25 minutes | **Servings:** 4

- 1-pound tilapia fillet
- 3 oz Parmesan, grated
- 1 tablespoon olive oil
- 1 teaspoon chili powder

1. Line the baking tray with baking paper.
2. Then rub the tilapia with olive oil and chili powder. Put it in the tray and top with Parmesan.
3. Bake the tilapia ta 365F for 25 minutes.

per serving: 194 calories, 28g protein, 1.1g carbohydrates, 9.2g fat, 0.2g fiber, 70mg cholesterol, 244mg sodium, 12mg potassium

Poached Salmon

Prep time: 10 minutes | **Cook time:** 20 minutes | **Servings:** 4

- ½ cup apples, chopped
- 1 cup of water
- 1-pound salmon fillet, chopped
- 1 tablespoon dried cilantro
- 1 teaspoon dried thyme

1. Pour water in the saucepan.
2. Add apples, salmon fillet, dried cilantro, and thyme.
3. Close the lid and cook the meal on medium heat for 20 minutes.

per serving: 165 calories, 22.1g protein, 4g carbohydrates, 7.1g fat, 0.8g fiber, 50mg cholesterol, 52mg sodium, 469mg potassium

Boiled Lobster Tails

Prep time: 10 minutes | **Cook time:** 15 minutes | **Servings:** 4

- 4 lobster tails, peeled
- 1 cup of water
- 1 tablespoon dried rosemary

1. Bring the water to boil.
2. Add dried rosemary and lobster tails. Cook the meal for 10 minutes on medium heat.

per serving: 79 calories, 16.2g protein, 0.5g carbohydrates, 0.8g fat, 0.4g fiber, 124mg cholesterol, 415mg sodium, 205mg potassium

Halibut Meatballs

Prep time: 10 minutes | **Cook time:** 10 minutes | **Servings:** 4

- 1-pound halibut fillet, minced
- 1 egg, beaten
- ½ cup almond flour
- 1 teaspoon dried rosemary
- 1 teaspoon dried basil
- ½ teaspoon ground turmeric
- 1 tablespoon olive oil

1. In the mixing bowl, mix halibut with egg, almond flour, dried rosemary, basil, and ground turmeric.
2. Make the meatballs.
3. Preheat the olive oil.
4. Put the meatballs in the olive oil and roast them for 3 minutes per side.

per serving: 512 calories, 33.7g protein, 3.2g carbohydrates, 39.5g fat, 1.7g fiber, 135mg cholesterol, 184mg sodium, 572mg potassium

Chili Salmon

Prep time: 10 minutes | **Cook time:** 12 minutes | **Servings:** 6

- 2-pounds salmon, fillet
- 2 chili peppers
- 1 tablespoon olive
- oil
- 1 sweet pepper, sliced

1. Preheat the olive oil in the skillet.
2. Add sweet peppers and chili pepper.
3. Roast the ingredients for 1 minute per side.
4. Then add salmon and cook it for 5 minutes per side on medium heat.

per serving: 227 calories, 29.6g protein, 1.6g carbohydrates, 11.7g fat, 0.3g fiber, 67mg cholesterol, 67mg sodium, 621mg potassium

Mayonnaise Salmon

Prep time: 10 minutes | **Cook time:** 10 minutes | **Servings:** 6

- 2-pounds salmon, chopped
- 2 tablespoons low-fat mayonnaise
- 1 teaspoon dried mint
- 1 teaspoon ground black pepper
- 2 tablespoons olive oil
- 1 tablespoon lemon juice

1. Preheat the olive oil well.
2. Then mix all remaining ingredients and put in the hot oil.
3. Cook the fish for 5 minutes per side.

per serving: 261 calories, 29.4g protein, 1.5g carbohydrates, 15.7g fat, 0.1g fiber, 68mg cholesterol, 102mg sodium, 590mg potassium

Turmeric Flounder

Prep time: 10 minutes | Cook time: 8 minutes | Servings: 4

- 1 tablespoon ground turmeric
- 1-pound flounder fillet, chopped
- ½ cup coconut

cream
- 1 teaspoon olive oil
- ½ teaspoon chili powder

1. Mix the flounder fillet with ground turmeric, coconut cream, and chili powder.
2. Preheat the olive oil well.
3. Put the fish mixture in the hot oil and cook it for 4 minutes per side.

per serving: 219 calories, 28.3g protein, 2.9g carbohydrates, 10.3g fat, 1.1g fiber, 77mg cholesterol, 128mg sodium, 518mg potassium

Parmesan Cod

Prep time: 10 minutes | Cook time: 10 minutes | Servings: 2

- 14 oz cod fillet
- 3 oz Parmesan, grated
- 1 teaspoon chili

powder
- 2 tablespoons olive oil

1. Preheat the olive oil.
2. Rub the cod fillet with chili powder and put in the olive oil.
3. Roast the fish for 2 minutes per side.
4. Then top the fish with parmesan, close the lid, and cook the meal for 5 minutes more.

per serving: 420 calories, 49.3g protein, 2.2g carbohydrates, 25.1g fat, 0.4g fiber, 83mg cholesterol, 532mg sodium, 25mg potassium

Coriander Salmon

Prep time: 10 minutes | Cook time: 15 minutes | Servings: 2

- 1-pound salmon fillet
- 1 tablespoon ground coriander

- 2 tablespoons olive oil
- 1 tablespoon apple cider vinegar

1. Mix the salmon fillet with ground coriander, olive oil, and apple cider vinegar.
2. Wrap the salmon in the foil and bake at 400F for 15 minutes.

per serving: 422 calories, 44g protein, 0.1g carbohydrates, 28g fat, 0g fiber, 100mg cholesterol, 101mg sodium, 879mg potassium

Seafood Fennel Stew

Prep time: 10 minutes | Cook time: 25 minutes | Servings: 6

- 1-pound fennel bulb, chopped
- 1-pound cod fillet, chopped
- 1 cup of water
- 1 teaspoon ground paprika

- ½ teaspoon ground turmeric
- 1 tablespoon olive oil
- 2 garlic cloves, diced

1. Pour olive oil in the skillet and add a fennel bulb. Roast it for 2 minutes per side.
2. Then add all remaining ingredients and stir the mixture.
3. Close the lid and cook the stew on medium heat for 20 minutes.

per serving: 107 calories, 14.6g protein, 6.2g carbohydrates, 3.2g fat, 2.5g fiber, 37mg cholesterol, 88mg sodium, 330mg potassium

Garlic Clams

Prep time: 10 minutes | Cook time: 10 minutes | Servings: 2

- 15 oz clams, cleaned
- 1 teaspoon minced garlic
- 1 tablespoon fresh

parsley, chopped
- 1 cup of water
- 1 tablespoon olive oil

1. Bring the water to the boil and put the clams inside. Boil them for 3 minutes.
2. Then preheat the olive oil well.
3. Put the cooked clams in the hot oil. Add minced garlic and parsley.
4. Stir the meal and cook it for 2-3 minutes.

per serving: 165 calories, 1.4g protein, 23.9g carbohydrates, 7.5g fat, 0.9g fiber, 0mg cholesterol, 775mg sodium, 207mg potassium

Salmon Cakes

Prep time: 10 minutes | Cook time: 15 minutes | Servings: 4

- 2 zucchinis, grated
- 1-pound salmon, minced
- 1 teaspoon ground black pepper
- ¼ cup almond flour
- 1 tablespoon olive oil

1. In the mixing bowl, mix zucchinis with salmon, ground black pepper, and almond flour.
2. Make the salmon cakes.
3. Line the baking tray with baking paper and put the salmon cakes inside.
4. Sprinkle them with olive oil and bake them at 365F for 15 minutes.

per serving: 239 calories, 24.8g protein, 5.1g carbohydrates, 14g fat, 2g fiber, 50mg cholesterol, 63mg sodium, 699mg potassium

Turmeric Salmon

Prep time: 10 minutes | Cook time: 10 minutes | Servings: 4

- 1-pound salmon fillet, chopped
- 1 teaspoon ground turmeric
- 1 teaspoon ground ginger
- 2 tablespoons olive oil

1. Mix salmon fillet with ground turmeric and ground ginger.
2. Preheat the olive oil in the skillet. Add salmon.
3. Roast the fish on medium heat for 4 minutes per side.

per serving: 214 calories, 22.1g protein, 0.7g carbohydrates, 14.1g fat, 0.2g fiber, 50mg cholesterol, 50mg sodium, 455mg potassium

Salmon Meatballs

Prep time: 15 minutes | Cook time: 6 minutes | Servings: 4

- 1-pound salmon fillet, minced
- 1 tablespoon minced garlic
- 2 tablespoons
- almond flour
- 1 teaspoon ground coriander
- 1 tablespoon olive oil

1. Mix salmon fillet with minced garlic, almond flour, and ground coriander.
2. Make the meatballs.
3. Preheat the skillet well, add olive oil.
4. Put the salmon meatballs in the hot oil and roast them for 3 minutes per side.

per serving: 204 calories, 22.9g protein, 1.4g carbohydrates, 12.2g fat, 0.4g fiber, 50mg cholesterol, 52mg sodium, 444mg potassium

Cod with Carrot

Prep time: 10 minutes | Cook time: 20 minutes | Servings: 2

- 16 oz salmon fillet, chopped
- 1 cup carrot, grated
- 1 tablespoon olive
- oil
- 1 teaspoon dried thyme
- ¼ cup of water

1. Mix olive oil with carrot and put it in the saucepan. Roast the mixture for 5 minutes.
2. Then add dried thyme, salmon, and water.
3. Cook the meal on medium heat for 15 minutes.

per serving: 384 calories, 44.5g protein, 5.7g carbohydrates, 21g fat, 1.5g fiber, 100mg cholesterol, 139mg sodium, 1051mg potassium

Ginger Scallops

Prep time: 10 minutes | Cook time: 5 minutes | Servings: 4

- 1-pound scallops
- 1 tablespoon minced ginger
- 2 tablespoons olive
- oil
- ½ teaspoon ground nutmeg

1. Rub the scallops with minced ginger and ground nutmeg,
2. Then preheat the olive oil well and add the scallops.
3. Roast them for 2 minutes per side or until they are light brown.

per serving: 166 calories, 19.2g protein, 3.8g carbohydrates, 8g fat, 0.2g fiber, 37mg cholesterol, 66mg sodium, 513mg potassium

Curry Trout

Prep time: 10 minutes | **Cook time:** 15 minutes | **Servings:** 4

- 1 cup of coconut milk
- 1 tablespoon curry paste
- 1-pound trout fillet, chopped
- 1 teaspoon olive oil

1. Preheat the olive oil well and put the trout inside. Roast it for 2 minutes per side.
2. Then mix coconut milk with curry paste.
3. Pour the liquid over the fish and close the lid. Cook the trout on medium heat for 10 minutes more.

per serving: 389 calories, 31.8g protein, 4.4g carbohydrates, 27.3g fat, 1.3g fiber, 84mg cholesterol, 85mg sodium, 683mg potassium

Tender Chives Salmon

Prep time: 10 minutes | **Cook time:** 5 minutes | **Servings:** 4

- 1-pound salmon fillet
- 2 oz chives, chopped
- 1 teaspoon ground turmeric
- 1 teaspoon chili powder
- 2 tablespoons olive oil

1. Rub the salmon fillet with ground turmeric, chili powder, and olive oil.
2. Put the fish in the well-preheat skillet and roast it for 2 minutes per side.
3. Then top the fish with chives and cook it for 1 minute more.

per serving: 218 calories, 22.6g protein, 1.3g carbohydrates, 14.3g fat, 0.7g fiber, 50mg cholesterol, 57mg sodium, 504mg potassium

Lemon Crab

Prep time: 10 minutes | **Cook time:** 6 minutes | **Servings:** 4

- 1-pound crab meat, chopped
- 1 lemon, chopped
- 1 tablespoon olive oil
- 1 teaspoon chili powder

1. Pour olive oil in the skillet. Preheat it well.
2. Add crab meat and roast it for 1 minute per side.
3. Then sprinkle the crab meat with chili powder and lemon juice and cook the meal on medium heat for 5 minutes more.

per serving: 138 calories, 14.4g protein, 3.7g carbohydrates, 5.7g fat, 0.6g fiber, 61mg cholesterol, 716mg sodium, 32mg potassium

Rosemary Salmon

Prep time: 10 minutes | **Cook time:** 6 minutes | **Servings:** 4

- 2-pounds salmon fillet, chopped
- 1 tablespoon dried rosemary
- 2 tablespoons olive oil

1. Preheat the grill to 400F.
2. Mix the salmon with rosemary and olive oil.
3. Put the fish pieces in the grill and cook them for 3 minutes per side.

per serving: 363 calories, 44g protein, 0.5g carbohydrates, 21.1g fat, 0.4g fiber, 100mg cholesterol, 100mg sodium, 879mg potassium

Garlic Salmon

Prep time: 10 minutes | **Cook time:** 10 minutes | **Servings:** 2

- 12 oz salmon fillet
- 1 tablespoon minced garlic
- 2 tablespoons olive oil
- 1 teaspoon dried dill

1. Rub the salmon fillet with minced garlic, olive oil, and dried dill.
2. Put the salmon in the well-preheated skillet and roast for 5 minutes per side.

per serving: 353 calories, 33.4g protein, 1.7g carbohydrates, 24.5g fat, 0.2g fiber, 75mg cholesterol, 77mg sodium, 687mg potassium

Thyme Haddock

Prep time: 10 minutes | **Cook time:** 10 minutes | **Servings:** 4

- 1-pound haddock fillets
- 1 tablespoon dried thyme
- 1 tablespoon olive oil
- 1 teaspoon lemon zest, grated

1. Mix fish with dried thyme, olive oil, and lemon zest.
2. Put the fish in the preheated to 400F grill and cook it for 4 minutes per side.

per serving: 159 calories, 27.6g protein, 0.5g carbohydrates, 4.6g fat, 0.3g fiber, 84mg cholesterol, 99mg sodium, 460mg potassium

Nutmeg Trout

Prep time: 10 minutes | **Cook time:** 10 minutes | **Servings:** 2

- 12 oz trout fillet
- 2 tablespoons olive oil
- 1 tablespoon
- lemon juice
- 1 teaspoon ground nutmeg

1. Rub the trout fillet with lemon juice and ground nutmeg.
2. Then brush it with olive oil and put it in the hot skillet.
3. Roast the fish for 5 minutes per side.

per serving: 451 calories, 45.4g protein, 0.7g carbohydrates, 28.9g fat, 0.3g fiber, 126mg cholesterol, 116mg sodium, 801mg potassium

Cayenne Pepper Shrimps

Prep time: 10 minutes | **Cook time:** 10 minutes | **Servings:** 5

- 2-pound shrimps, peeled
- 1 tablespoon cayenne pepper
- 2 tablespoon lemon juice
- 1 tablespoon olive oil

1. Mix shrimps with olive oil, lemon juice, and cayenne pepper.
2. Preheat the skillet well and put the shrimps inside.
3. Cook them for 3 minutes per side.

per serving: 244 calories, 41.5g protein, 3.5g carbohydrates, 6.1g fat, 0.3g fiber,382mg cholesterol, 444mg sodium, 336mg potassium

Tomato Calamari

Prep time: 10 minutes | **Cook time:** 15 minutes | **Servings:** 6

- 2-pound calamari, sliced
- 1 cup tomatoes
- 1 chili pepper,
- chopped
- 2 tablespoons olive oil

1. Mix olive oil with chopped tomatoes and put them in the saucepan.
2. Roast the mixture for 5 minutes.
3. Add chili pepper and calamari. Carefully mix the ingredients.
4. Close the lid and cook the seafood for 10 minutes.

per serving: 188 calories, 10.9g protein, 12.6g carbohydrates, 10.1g fat, 1.1g fiber, 0mg cholesterol, 341mg sodium, 73mg potassium

Oregano Mackerel

Prep time: 10 minutes | **Cook time:** 10 minutes | **Servings:** 4

- 1-pound mackerel fillet, chopped
- 2 tablespoons
- dried oregano
- 1 tablespoon olive oil

1. Preheat the oil in the skillet well.
2. Rub the mackerel with dried oregano and put it in the hot oil.
3. Roast it for 4 minutes per side.

per serving: 334 calories, 27.3g protein, 1.5g carbohydrates, 23.9g fat, 1g fiber, 85mg cholesterol, 94mg sodium, 492mg potassium

Baked Salmon

Prep time: 10 minutes | **Cook time:** 20 minutes | **Servings:** 4

- 1-pound salmon fillet
- 2 tablespoons olive oil
- 1 tablespoon
- ground black pepper
- 1 teaspoon chili powder

1. Rub the salmon fillet with olive oil, ground black pepper, and chili powder.
2. Put the fish in the tray and bake at 375F for 20 minutes.

per serving: 216 calories, 22.3g protein, 1.4g carbohydrates, 14.2g fat, 0.6g fiber, 50mg cholesterol, 57mg sodium, 468mg potassium

Cod Stew

Prep time: 10 minutes | **Cook time:** 25 minutes | **Servings:** 4

- 2 cups green peas, frozen
- 1-pound cod fillet, chopped
- 1 cup of water
- 1 onion, sliced
- 1 teaspoon dried rosemary
- 1 teaspoon chili powder

1. Put all ingredients in the saucepan and gently mix.
2. Close the lid and cook the stew on medium heat for 25 minutes.

per serving: 164 calories, 24.6g protein, 13.6g carbohydrates, 1.5g fat, 4.6g fiber, 56mg cholesterol, 84mg sodium, 233mg potassium

Fried Scallops

Prep time: 10 minutes | **Cook time:** 5 minutes | **Servings:** 4

- 1-pound scallops
- 3 tablespoons olive oil
- 1 tablespoon
- lemon juice
- 1 teaspoon minced garlic

1. Rub the scallops with olive oil, lemon juice, and minced garlic.
2. Then preheat the skillet well and put the scallops inside.
3. Roast them for 2 minutes per side.

per serving: 192 calories, 19.1g protein, 3g carbohydrates, 11.4g fat, 0g fiber, 3mg cholesterol, 183mg sodium, 373mg potassium

Lime Mackerel

Prep time: 10 minutes | **Cook time:** 25 minutes | **Servings:** 4

- 1 lime
- 1-pound mackerel fillet, chopped
- 1 teaspoon ground
- ginger
- ¼ cup of water
- 1 teaspoon olive oil

1. Preheat the oil well.
2. Add mackerel and ground ginger.
3. Cook the fish for 1 minute per side.
4. Add water and juice from 1 lime.
5. Close the lid and cook the fish for 15 minutes.

per serving: 314 calories, 27.2g protein, 2.1g carbohydrates, 21.4g fat, 0.5g fiber, 85mg cholesterol, 95mg sodium, 478mg potassium

Curry Tilapia

Prep time: 10 minutes | **Cook time:** 15 minutes | **Servings:** 2

- 14 oz tilapia fillet, chopped
- 1 teaspoon curry powder
- ½ cup of coconut milk
- 1 teaspoon olive oil

1. Pour olive oil in the skillet and preheat it well.
2. Add tilapia and cook it for 1 minute per side.
3. Meanwhile, mix coconut milk with curry powder.
4. Pour the mixture over the fish and cook the meal for 10 minutes more.

per serving: 325 calories, 38.4g protein, 3.9g carbohydrates, 18.6g fat, 1.7g fiber, 97mg cholesterol, 80mg sodium, 173mg potassium

Garlic Tuna

Prep time: 10 minutes | **Cook time:** 15 minutes | **Servings:** 4

- 1-pound tuna fillet, chopped
- 1 teaspoon minced garlic
- 1 tablespoon olive oil
- ½ cup plain yogurt
- ¼ cup of water

1. Pour olive oil in the skillet.
2. Add minced garlic and tuna. Roast the ingredients for 2 minutes per side.
3. Then add plain yogurt and water.
4. Close the lid and cook the fish for 10 minutes more.

per serving: 264 calories, 31.9g protein, 2.4g carbohydrates, 13.9g fat, 0g fiber, 37mg cholesterol,79mg sodium, 452mg potassium

Tomato Mackerel

Prep time: 10 minutes | **Cook time:** 25 minutes | **Servings:** 4

- 1 cup tomatoes, chopped
- 1 cup onion, chopped
- 1-pound mackerel,
- chopped
- 1 teaspoon peppercorns
- 1 cup of water

1. Pour water in the saucepan.
2. Add peppercorns, onion, and tomatoes.
3. Bring the mixture to boil and add mackerel. Close the lid and cook the meal for 15 minutes more.

per serving: 318 calories, 27.8g protein, 4.8g carbohydrates, 20.3g fat, 1.3g fiber, 85mg cholesterol, 99mg sodium, 611mg potassium

Jalapeno Snapper

Prep time: 10 minutes | **Cook time:** 20 minutes | **Servings:** 2

- 16 oz red snapper fillets, boneless and skinless
- 2 jalapenos, sliced
- 1 tablespoon olive oil
- 1 lemon, chopped
- ¼ cup of water

1. Preheat the olive oil in the skillet.
2. Add fish, lemon, and jalapenos.
3. Cook the mixture for 4 minutes per side.
4. Add water and close the lid.
5. Cook the snapper on medium heat for 10 minutes.

per serving: 363 calories, 60.2g protein, 3.5g carbohydrates, 11.1g fat, 1.2g fiber, 107mg cholesterol, 131mg sodium, 1254mg potassium

Lemongrass Mackerel

Prep time: 10 minutes | **Cook time:** 25 minutes | **Servings:** 4

- 1-pound mackerel fillet
- 1 tablespoon lemongrass, chopped
- 1 cup coconut cream
- ½ teaspoon ground clove

1. Rub the mackerel fillet with lemongrass and ground clove.
2. Put the fish in the tray and top with lemongrass.
3. Bake it at 365F for 25 minutes.

per serving: 437 calories, 28.5g protein, 3.8g carbohydrates, 34.6g fat, 1.4g fiber, 85mg cholesterol, 104mg sodium, 624mg potassium

Stuffed Peppers with Cod

Prep time: 10 minutes | **Cook time:** 25 minutes | **Servings:** 4

- 10 oz cod fillet, minced
- 1 onion, minced
- 1 teaspoon ground black pepper
- 4 bell peppers, trimmed, seeded
- ¼ cup coconut cream
- 1 teaspoon olive oil

1. Mix cod with onion and ground black pepper.
2. Then fill the peppers with the cod mixture and put it in the saucepan.
3. Add olive oil and coconut cream. Close the lid.
4. Cook the meal on medium heat for 25 minutes.

per serving: 152 calories, 14.6g protein, 12.7g carbohydrates, 5.7g fat, 2.7g fiber, 35mg cholesterol, 51mg sodium, 310mg potassium

Salmon and Carrot Balls

Prep time: 10 minutes | **Cook time:** 8 minutes | **Servings:** 4

- 1-pound salmon fillet, minced
- ¼ cup carrot, grated
- 3 tablespoons almond flour
- 1 egg, beaten
- 1 teaspoon ground coriander
- ½ teaspoon minced garlic
- 2 tablespoons olive oil

1. In the mixing bowl, mix salmon with carrot, almond flour, egg, ground coriander, and minced garlic.
2. Make the balls.
3. Preheat the olive oil well.
4. Put the fish balls in the hot oil and roast them for 4 minutes per side.

per serving: 261 calories, 24.6g protein, 2g carbohydrates, 17.6g fat, 0.7g fiber, 91mg cholesterol, 72mg sodium, 474mg potassium

Scallop Stew

Prep time: 10 minutes | **Cook time:** 15 minutes | **Servings:** 4

- 1 pound scallops
- 2 tablespoons olive oil
- 1 teaspoon Italian seasonings
- ½ cup of water
- 1 cup carrot, grated

1. Pour olive oil in the saucepan and preheat it.
2. Add carrot and cook it for 3 minutes per side.
3. Then add Italian seasonings, scallops, and water.
4. Close the lid and cook the stew for 10 minutes on medium heat.

per serving: 175 calories, 19.3g protein, 5.5g carbohydrates, 8.2g fat, 0.7g fiber, 38mg cholesterol, 203mg sodium, 454mg potassium

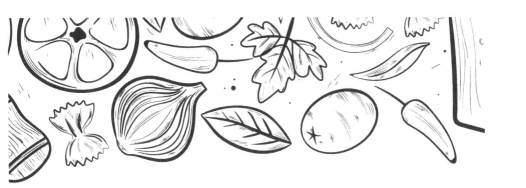

Vegan &
Vegetarian

Cauliflower Steaks

Prep time: 10 minutes | **Cook time:** 40 minutes | **Servings:** 6

- 2-pounds cauliflower head
- 2 tablespoons olive oil
- 1 teaspoon ground turmeric
- 1 oz Parmesan, grated

1. Slice the cauliflower head into the steaks and rub with ground turmeric and olive oil.
2. Then put the cauliflower steaks in the tray and top with Parmesan.
3. Bake the cauliflower steaks at 360F for 40 minutes.

per serving: 94 calories, 4.5g protein, 8.4g carbohydrates, 5.9g fat, 3.9g fiber, 3mg cholesterol, 89mg sodium, 467mg potassium

Jalapeno Corn

Prep time: 10 minutes | **Cook time:** 15 minutes | **Servings:** 4

- 2 cups corn kernels
- 2 jalapenos, sliced
- ½ cup coconut cream

1. Put all ingredients in the baking pan and carefully mix.
2. Bake the meal at 360F for 15 minutes.

per serving: 137 calories, 3.3g protein, 16.6g carbohydrates, 8.1g fat, 3g fiber, 3mg cholesterol, 16mg sodium, 302mg potassium

Vegetable Roast

Prep time: 10 minutes | **Cook time:** 25 minutes | **Servings:** 4

- 1 cup Brussel sprouts
- 1 cup carrot, chopped
- 1 onion, chopped
- 1 teaspoon dried parsley
- ½ teaspoon ground coriander
- 2 tablespoons olive oil
- 2 garlic cloves, peeled, crushed

1. Put all ingredients in the baking tray and carefully mix.
2. Cook the meal at 400F for 25 minutes. Flip the vegetables on another side after 15 minutes of cooking.

per serving: 94 calories, 1.4g protein, 7.8g carbohydrates, 7.1g fat, 2.1g fiber, 0mg cholesterol, 26mg sodium, 222mg potassium

Corn Bake

Prep time: 10 minutes | **Cook time:** 20 minutes | **Servings:** 4

- 2 cups corn kernels
- 4 oz Parmesan, grated
- ¼ cup coconut
- cream
- 1 teaspoon dried basil

1. In the mixing bowl, mix corn kernels with coconut cream, and dried basil.
2. Put the mixture in the baking pan and top with Parmesan.
3. Bake the corn bake at 360F for 20 minutes.

per serving: 192 calories, 12g protein, 16.4g carbohydrates, 10.6g fat, 2.4g fiber, 20mg cholesterol, 277mg sodium, 248mg potassium

Thyme Carrots

Prep time: 10 minutes | **Cook time:** 40 minutes | **Servings:** 4

- 8 carrots, peeled
- 1 tablespoons dried thyme
- 2 tablespoons
- lemon juice
- 2 tablespoons olive oil

1. In the shallow bowl, mix dried thyme with lemon juice and olive oil.
2. Then place the carrots in the tray and sprinkle with thyme mixture.
3. Bake the carrot at 360F for 40 minutes.

per serving: 114 calories, 1.1g protein, 12.6g carbohydrates, 7.1g fat, 3.3g fiber, 0mg cholesterol, 86mg sodium, 405mg potassium

Baked Squash

Prep time: 10 minutes | **Cook time:** 25 minutes | **Servings:** 4

- 4 zucchinis, halved
- 1 tablespoon olive oil
- 1 teaspoon dried
- thyme
- ½ teaspoon cayenne pepper

1. Sprinkle the zucchinis with olive oil, dried thyme, and cayenne pepper.
2. Put the zucchini halves in the tray and bake at 400F for 25 minutes.

per serving: 63 calories, 2.4g protein, 6.9g carbohydrates, 3.9g fat, 2.3g fiber, 0mg cholesterol, 20mg sodium, 520mg potassium

Cinnamon Pumpkin Cubes

Prep time: 10 minutes | **Cook time:** 50 minutes | **Servings:** 4

- 1 teaspoon ground cinnamon
- 2 cups pumpkin, chopped
- 1 tablespoon olive oil
- 1 teaspoon dried basil

1. Mix ground cinnamon with pumpkin, and dried basil.
2. Then put the pumpkin in the tray and sprinkle with olive oil.
3. Cook the pumpkin at 350F for 50 minutes in the oven.

per serving: 73 calories, 1.4g protein, 10.4g carbohydrates, 3.9g fat, 3.9g fiber, 0mg cholesterol, 6mg sodium, 256mg potassium

Spicy Daikon Radish

Prep time: 10 minutes | **Cook time:** 0 minutes | **Servings:** 6

- 1-pound daikon radish, peeled, chopped
- 2 cucumbers, chopped
- 2 oz chives, chopped
- 1/3 cup plain yogurt

1. Put all ingredients in the mixing bowl.
2. Carefully mix the meal and transfer in the serving bowls.

per serving: 43 calories, 3.2g protein, 8g carbohydrates, 0.4g fat, 2.3g fiber, 1mg cholesterol, 27mg sodium, 381mg potassium

Radish Roast

Prep time: 5 minutes | **Cook time:** 20 minutes | **Servings:** 4

- 4 cups radish, halved
- 1 teaspoon dried rosemary
- 3 tablespoons olive oil

1. Line the baking tray with baking paper and put radish inside.
2. Sprinkle it with dried rosemary and olive oil.
3. Bake the radish at 360F for 20 minutes.

per serving: 110 calories, 0.8g protein, 4.1g carbohydrates, 10.7g fat, 2g fiber, 0mg cholesterol, 45mg sodium, 273mg potassium

Mint Green Beans

Prep time: 10 minutes | **Cook time:** 20 minutes | **Servings:** 4

- 1-pound green beans, trimmed, chopped
- 1 teaspoon dried mint
- 1 tablespoon olive oil
- 1 teaspoon chili flakes

1. Put the green beans in the mixing bowl.
2. Add dried mint, olive oil, and chili flakes. Shake the mixture well.
3. Then transfer it in the baking tray and bake at 365F for 20 minutes.

per serving: 65 calories, 2.1g protein, 8.2g carbohydrates, 3.6g fat, 3.9g fiber, 0mg cholesterol, 7mg sodium, 240mg potassium

Marinated Collard Greens

Prep time: 20 minutes | **Cook time:** 0 minutes | **Servings:** 4

- 10 oz collard greens, chopped
- 3 tablespoons lemon juice
- 1 teaspoon minced garlic
- ½ teaspoon minced ginger
- 2 tablespoons olive oil

1. In the mixing bowl, mix lemon juice with minced garlic, minced ginger, and olive oil.
2. Then add collard greens and carefully mix the mixture.
3. Leave the meal for 10 minutes to marinate.

per serving: 84 calories, 1.7g protein, 4.5g carbohydrates, 7.6g fat, 2.4g fiber, 0mg cholesterol, 14mg sodium, 20mg potassium

Parmesan Kale

Prep time: 5 minutes | **Cook time:** 20 minutes | **Servings:** 4

- 4 cups kale, roughly chopped
- 2 oz Parmesan, grated
- 1 tablespoon olive oil

1. Put the kale in the tray and flatten it well.
2. Then sprinkle the kale with olive oil and Parmesan.
3. Cook the kale at 350F for 20 minutes.

per serving: 109 calories, 6.6g protein, 7.5g carbohydrates, 6.5g fat, 1g fiber, 10mg cholesterol, 161mg sodium, 329mg potassium

Carrot Noodles

Prep time: 15 minutes | **Cook time:** 0 minutes | **Servings:** 6

- 6 carrots, spiralized
- 1 tablespoon olive oil
- 1 teaspoon dried cilantro
- ¼ teaspoon dried rosemary

1. In the bowl, mix carrots with olive oil, dried cilantro, and rosemary.
2. Carefully mix the meal and leave for 5-7 minutes to marinate.

per serving: 45 calories, 0.5g protein, 6g carbohydrates, 2.3g fat, 1.5g fiber, 0mg cholesterol, 42mg sodium, 196mg potassium

Garlic Green Beans

Prep time: 10 minutes | **Cook time:** 30 minutes | **Servings:** 4

- 2 pounds green beans, trimmed
- 2 tablespoons olive oil
- 1 tablespoon minced garlic
- 1 teaspoon dried cilantro

1. Mix green beans with olive oil, minced garlic, and dried oregano.
2. Then line the baking tray with baking paper.
3. Put the green beans inside the tray, flatten them, and bake at 360F for 30 minutes. Flip the green beans on another side after 15 minutes of cooking.

per serving: 133 calories, 4.3g protein, 16.9g carbohydrates, 7.3g fat, 7.8g fiber, 0mg cholesterol, 14mg sodium, 483mg potassium

Chickpeas Spread

Prep time: 10 minutes | **Cook time:** 0 minutes | **Servings:** 3

- 1 cup chickpeas, cooked
- 1 tablespoon tahini paste
- 2 tablespoons lemon juice
- ¼ cup olive oil

1. Put all ingredients in the blender.
2. Blend the mixture until smooth.
3. Transfer it in the serving bowl.

per serving: 419 calories, 13.8g protein, 41.7g carbohydrates, 23.6g fat, 12.1g fiber, 0mg cholesterol, 24mg sodium, 617mg potassium

Creamy Spinach

Prep time: 10 minutes | **Cook time:** 12 minutes | **Servings:** 4

- 4 cups spinach, chopped
- 1 cup coconut cream
- ½ teaspoon
- cayenne pepper
- ½ teaspoon ground nutmeg
- 2 oz Parmesan, grated

1. Put all ingredients in the saucepan and carefully mix.
2. Close the lid and simmer the meal on medium heat for 12 minutes.

per serving: 193 calories, 6.8g protein, 5.2g carbohydrates, 17.6g fat, 2.1g fiber, 10mg cholesterol, 164mg sodium, 331mg potassium

Eggplant Rings

Prep time: 10 minutes | **Cook time:** 15 minutes | **Servings:** 4

- 3 eggplants, sliced
- 2 tablespoons minced garlic
- ¼ cup plain yogurt
- 1 tablespoon olive oil

1. Preheat the skillet well.
2. Then add olive oil.
3. Put the sliced eggplants in the skillet in one layer and roast them for 2 minutes per side.
4. Then mix plain yogurt with minced garlic.
5. Top the eggplants with plain yogurt mixture.

per serving: 150 calories, 5.2g protein, 26.6g carbohydrates, 4.5g fat, 14.6g fiber, 1mg cholesterol, 20mg sodium, 994mg potassium

Baked Jalapenos

Prep time: 10 minutes | **Cook time:** 20 minutes | **Servings:** 4

- 8 jalapenos, trimmed
- 1 tablespoon olive
- oil
- 1 teaspoon fennel seeds

1. Line the baking tray with baking paper.
2. Then put the jalapenos in the baking tray and sprinkle with olive oil and fennel seeds.
3. Bake the jalapenos at 375F for 20 minutes.

per serving: 40 calories, 0.5g protein, 1.9g carbohydrates, 3.7g fat, 1g fiber, 0mg cholesterol, 1mg sodium, 69mg potassium

Baked Leek

Prep time: 10 minutes | **Cook time:** 20 minutes | **Servings:** 4

- 1-pound leek, sliced
- 1 carrot, grated
- 1 cup of coconut milk
- 1 teaspoon olive oil
- 1 teaspoon ground black pepper

1. Mix leek with grated carrot, olive oil, ground black pepper, and coconut milk.
2. Put the mixture in the baking pan and flatten it gently.
3. Bake the meal at 365F for 20 minutes.

per serving: 225 calories, 3.3g protein, 21.2g carbohydrates, 15.8g fat, 3.9g fiber, 0mg cholesterol, 42mg sodium, 417mg potassium

Broccoli Steaks

Prep time: 10 minutes | **Cook time:** 20 minutes | **Servings:** 4

- 1-pound broccoli head
- 1 teaspoon
- cayenne pepper
- 2 tablespoons olive oil

1. Slice the broccoli head into the steaks and put in the baking tray in one layer.
2. Sprinkle the vegetables with cayenne pepper and olive oil.
3. Bake the broccoli steaks at 365F for 10 minutes per side.

per serving: 100 calories, 3.2g protein, 7.8g carbohydrates, 7.5g fat, 3.1g fiber, 0mg cholesterol, 38mg sodium, 368mg potassium

Baked Eggplants

Prep time: 10 minutes | **Cook time:** 30 minutes | **Servings:** 4

- 4 eggplants, halved
- 1 teaspoon minced
- garlic
- 2 tablespoons olive oil

1. Rub the eggplants with minced garlic and olive oil.
2. Put the eggplant halves in the tray and bake at 375F for 30 minutes.

per serving: 198 calories, 5.4g protein, 32.5g carbohydrates, 8g fat, 19.4g fiber, 0mg cholesterol, 11mg sodium, 1258mg potassium

Lemon Bok Choy

Prep time: 10 minutes | **Cook time:** 20 minutes | **Servings:** 4

- 1 pound bok choy, sliced
- 1 lemon
- 1 tablespoon olive
- oil
- 1 teaspoon cumin seeds

1. Preheat the olive oil in the skillet well.
2. Add bok choy and roast it for 1 minute per side.
3. Then sprinkle the bok choy with cumin seeds.
4. Squeeze the lemon juice over the bok choy, carefully mix the meal, and cook it on low heat for 15 minutes.

per serving: 51 calories, 2g protein, 4.1g carbohydrates, 3.9g fat, 1.6g fiber, 0mg cholesterol, 75mg sodium, 315mg potassium

Curry Tofu

Prep time: 20 minutes | **Cook time:** 5 minutes | **Servings:** 4

- 1-pound tofu, cubed
- 1 teaspoon curry powder
- 1 tablespoon olive
- oil
- ½ cup coconut cream
- 1 teaspoon lemon zest, grated

1. In the mixing bowl, mix curry powder with olive oil, coconut cream, and lemon zest.
2. Then add tofu and mix well.
3. Leave the mixture for 10 minutes to marinate.
4. Then preheat the skillet well.
5. Add tofu and cook it for 2 minutes per side.

per serving: 180 calories, 10.1g protein, 4g carbohydrates, 15.5g fat, 1.9g fiber, 0mg cholesterol, 18mg sodium, 256mg potassium

Cumin Zucchini Rings

Prep time: 10 minutes | **Cook time:** 15 minutes | **Servings:** 5

- 3 zucchinis, sliced
- 1 tablespoon cumin seeds
- 1 tablespoon olive
- oil
- ¼ teaspoon cayenne pepper

1. Line the baking tray with baking paper.
2. Put the zucchini slices inside the baking tray in one layer.
3. Then sprinkle them with cumin seeds, olive oil, and cayenne pepper.
4. Bake the zucchini rings for 15 minutes at 360F.

per serving: 48 calories, 1.6g protein, 4.5g carbohydrates, 3.3g fat, 1.4g fiber, 0mg cholesterol, 14mg sodium, 331mg potassium

Mushroom Caps

Prep time: 10 minutes | **Cook time:** 20 minutes | **Servings:** 5

- 5 Portobello mushrooms (caps)
- 3 oz tofu, shredded
- ½ teaspoon curry paste
- 2 tablespoons coconut cream
- 1 teaspoon olive oil

1. In the mixing bowl, mix curry powder with coconut cream, olive oil, and shredded tofu.
2. Then fill the mushrooms with the shredded tofu mixture and put in the tray in one layer.
3. Bake the mushrooms at 360F for 20 minutes.

per serving: 57 calories, 4.6g protein, 3.8g carbohydrates, 3.4g fat, 1.3g fiber, 0mg cholesterol, 3mg sodium, 341mg potassium

Ginger Baked Mango

Prep time: 10 minutes | **Cook time:** 20 minutes | **Servings:** 4

- 2 mangos, pitted, halved
- 1 teaspoon minced ginger
- 1 tablespoon olive oil
- ¼ teaspoon dried rosemary

1. Put the mango halves in the baking tray and sprinkle with olive oil.
2. Then sprinkle the fruit with minced ginger and dried rosemary.
3. Bake the mango at 360F for 20 minutes.

per serving: 133 calories, 1.4g protein, 25.5g carbohydrates, 4.2g fat, 2.8g fiber, 0mg cholesterol, 2mg sodium, 289mg potassium

Poached Green Beans

Prep time: 10 minutes | **Cook time:** 15 minutes | **Servings:** 4

- 1-pound green beans, trimmed
- 2 cups of water
- 1 garlic clove, diced
- 2 tablespoons olive oil
- 1 tablespoon lime juice

1. Bring the water to boil and add green beans. Boil them for 10 minutes.
2. Then remove the green beans from water and mix with garlic clove, olive oil, and lime juice.

per serving: 97 calories, 2.1g protein, 8.6g carbohydrates, 7.2g fat, 3.9g fiber, 0mg cholesterol, 11mg sodium, 244mg potassium

Baked Avocado

Prep time: 10 minutes | **Cook time:** 20 minutes | **Servings:** 4

- 2 avocados, peeled, pitted, halved
- 1 tablespoon olive oil
- ½ teaspoon dried thyme

1. Put the avocado halves in the baking tray and sprinkle with olive oil and dried thyme.
2. Bake the avocados at 365F for 120 minutes.

per serving: 235 calories, 1.9g protein, 8.7g carbohydrates, 23.1g fat, 6.8g fiber, 0mg cholesterol, 6mg sodium, 488mg potassium

Green Peas Paste

Prep time: 10 minutes | **Cook time:** 0 minutes | **Servings:** 4

- 2 cups green peas, boiled
- 1 tablespoon almond butter
- ¼ cup fresh parsley, chopped
- 2 tablespoons lemon juice

1. Put all ingredients in the blender and blend until smooth.
2. Transfer the mixture into the serving bowl.

per serving: 86 calories, 5g protein, 11.6g carbohydrates, 2.6g fat, 4.3g fiber, 0mg cholesterol, 8mg sodium, 237mg potassium

Baked Cremini Mushrooms

Prep time: 10 minutes | **Cook time:** 30 minutes | **Servings:** 4

- 3 cups cremini mushrooms
- ¼ cup plain yogurt
- ¼ cup fresh parsley, chopped
- 1 teaspoon minced garlic
- 1 teaspoon ground turmeric
- 1 tablespoon olive oil

1. Mix cremini mushrooms with plain yogurt, parsley, and all remaining ingredients.
2. Put the mixture in the tray and bake at 350F for 30 minutes.

per serving: 60 calories, 2.4g protein, 4.1g carbohydrates, 3.8g fat, 0.6g fiber, 1mg cholesterol, 16mg sodium, 315mg potassium

Bean Spread

Prep time: 10 minutes | **Cook time:** 0 minutes | **Servings:** 6

- 2 cups red kidney beans, boiled
- 3 tablespoons plain yogurt
- 1 teaspoon ground nutmeg
- 1 teaspoon cayenne pepper
- 1 tablespoon fresh cilantro, chopped

1. Blend the red kidney beans until you get a smooth paste.
2. Then mix the beans with plain yogurt, ground nutmeg, cayenne pepper, and cilantro.
3. Carefully mix the spread.

per serving: 215 calories, 14.3g protein, 38.5g carbohydrates, 0.9g fat, 9.5g fiber, 0mg cholesterol, 13mg sodium, 860mg potassium

Baked Garlic

Prep time: 10 minutes | **Cook time:** 30 minutes | **Servings:** 4

- 8 oz garlic cloves, peeled
- 2 tablespoons olive oil
- 1 teaspoon dried rosemary

1. Put the garlic cloves in the tray and sprinkle with olive oil and dried rosemary.
2. Bake the garlic at 350F for 30 minutes.

per serving: 145 calories, 3.6g protein, 18.9g carbohydrates, 7.3g fat, 1.3g fiber, 0mg cholesterol, 10mg sodium, 230mg potassium

Eggplant Balls

Prep time: 10 minutes | **Cook time:** 5 minutes | **Servings:** 6

- 2 cups eggplants, peeled, boiled
- ½ cup almond flour
- 1 teaspoon ground cumin
- ½ teaspoon ground coriander
- 1 teaspoon chili powder
- 1 tablespoon olive oil

1. Blend the eggplant until smooth and mix it with almond flour, ground cumin, ground coriander, and chili powder.
2. Make the small balls.
3. After this, preheat the olive oil in the skillet well.
4. Put the eggplant balls inside and roast them for 2 minutes per side.

per serving: 86 calories, 2.4g protein, 4g carbohydrates, 7g fat, 2.2g fiber, 0mg cholesterol, 9mg sodium, 77mg potassium

Spicy Artichoke

Prep time: 10 minutes | **Cook time:** 35 minutes | **Servings:** 2

- 2 artichokes, halved
- 1 teaspoon minced garlic
- ½ teaspoon ground coriander
- ¼ teaspoon dried thyme
- 1 teaspoon dried oregano
- 4 teaspoons olive oil

1. Put the artichokes in the tray.
2. Then rub them with minced garlic, ground coriander, dried thyme, and oregano.
3. Sprinkle the artichokes with olive oil and cook them at 350F for 35 minutes.

per serving: 161 calories, 5.5g protein, 18.1g carbohydrates, 9.7g fat, 9.2g fiber, 0mg cholesterol, 153mg sodium, 619mg potassium

Baked Turnip

Prep time: 10 minutes | **Cook time:** 35 minutes | **Servings:** 3

- 2 cups turnips, peeled, roughly chopped
- 1 tablespoon olive
- oil
- 1 teaspoon dried oregano

1. Put the turnip in the baking tray and flatten it gently.
2. Sprinkle the vegetables with olive oil and dried oregano.
3. Bake the turnip at 355F for 35 minutes.

per serving: 65 calories, 0.7g protein, 5.7g carbohydrates, 4.7g fat, 1.5g fiber, 0mg cholesterol, 53mg sodium, 162mg potassium

Mushrooms Cakes

Prep time: 10 minutes | **Cook time:** 10 minutes | **Servings:** 8

- 3 cups mushrooms, sliced
- ½ cup almond flour
- 1 teaspoon chili flakes
- 1 teaspoon ground coriander
- 1 tablespoon olive oil
- ¼ cup plain yogurt

1. In the mixing bowl, mix sliced mushrooms with almond flour, chili flakes, ground coriander, and yogurt.
2. Then preheat the olive oil well in the skillet.
3. Make the small cakes from the mushroom mixture and put in the hot skillet.
4. Roast the mushroom cakes for 4 minutes per side.

per serving: 68 calories, 2.8g protein, 2.9g carbohydrates, 5.3g fat, 1g fiber, 0mg cholesterol, 9mg sodium, 102mg potassium

Baked Grapes

Prep time: 10 minutes | **Cook time:** 20 minutes | **Servings:** 6

- 3 cups green grapes
- 1 oz raisins, chopped
- 1 tablespoon olive
- oil
- 1 tablespoon lemon juice
- 1 teaspoon dried oregano

1. Mix grapes with raisins, olive oil, lemon juice, and dried oregano.
2. Put the mixture in the tray and bake at 360F for 20 minutes.

per serving: 66 calories, 0.5g protein, 11.8g carbohydrates, 2.6g fat, 0.7g fiber, 0mg cholesterol, 2mg sodium, 131mg potassium

Baked Butternut Squash

Prep time: 10 minutes | **Cook time:** 35 minutes | **Servings:** 4

- 1-pound butternut squash, chopped
- 1 teaspoon ground ginger
- 1 teaspoon ground paprika
- 1 tablespoon olive oil

1. In the mixing bowl mix butternut squash with ground ginger, paprika, and olive oil.
2. Put the butternut squash mixture in the tray, flatten it well and bake at 360F for 35 minutes.

per serving: 84 calories, 1.3g protein, 13.9g carbohydrates, 3.7g fat, 2.5g fiber, 0mg cholesterol, 5mg sodium, 418mg potassium

Cauliflower Balls

Prep time: 10 minutes | **Cook time:** 16 minutes | **Servings:** 4

- 2 cups cauliflower, shredded
- 3 oz tofu, shredded
- 3 tablespoons almond flour
- 2 tablespoons
- coconut cream
- 1 teaspoon curry powder
- 1 tablespoon olive oil

1. In the mixing bowl, mix shredded cauliflower with tofu, almond flour, coconut cream, and curry powder.
2. Make the balls from the mixture.
3. Then preheat the skillet well.
4. Add olive oil.
5. Then add cauliflower balls in the hot oil and roast them for 4 minutes per side or until the balls are light brown.

per serving: 108 calories, 4.1g protein, 4.9g carbohydrates, 8.8g fat, 2.3g fiber, 0mg cholesterol, 21mg sodium, 210mg potassium

Zucchini Cakes

Prep time: 10 minutes | **Cook time:** 15 minutes | **Servings:** 4

- 2 zucchinis, grated
- 3 tablespoons almond flour
- 1 teaspoon ground
- coriander
- 1 tablespoon olive oil

1. In the mixing bowl, mix grated zucchini with almond flour and ground coriander.
2. Preheat the skillet and pour the olive oil inside.
3. Preheat the oil.
4. Then make the cakes from the zucchini mixture and put them in the hot oil.
5. Cook the zucchini cakes for 3-4 minutes per side.

per serving: 77 calories, 2.3g protein, 4.4g carbohydrates, 6.2g fat, 1.6g fiber, 0mg cholesterol, 12mg sodium, 257mg potassium

Baked Onions

Prep time: 10 minutes | **Cook time:** 20 minutes | **Servings:** 4

- 4 red onions, peeled
- 1 teaspoon dried dill
- 1 teaspoon garlic powder
- 2 tablespoons olive oil

1. Make the cuts in the onions and sprinkle them with dried dill, garlic powder, and olive oil.
2. Then wrap the onions in the foil and put in the tray.
3. Bake the onions at 400F for 20 minutes.

per serving: 107 calories, 1.4g protein, 10.9g carbohydrates, 7.1g fat, 2.5g fiber, 0mg cholesterol, 5mg sodium, 177mg potassium

Mushroom Steaks

Prep time: 10 minutes | **Cook time:** 10 minutes | **Servings:** 2

- 2 Portobello mushrooms
- 1 tablespoon olive oil
- ½ teaspoon ground black pepper

1. Beat the mushrooms gently with the help of the kitchen hammer.
2. Then sprinkle the mushroom steaks with ground black pepper and olive oil.
3. Roast the mushrooms steaks in the well-preheat skillet for 5 minutes per side.

per serving: 81 calories, 3.1g protein, 3.3g carbohydrates, 7g fat, 1.1g fiber, 0mg cholesterol, 0mg sodium, 307mg potassium

Avocado Spread

Prep time: 10 minutes | **Cook time:** 0 minutes | **Servings:** 2

- 1 avocado, pitted, chopped, peeled
- ¼ cup plain yogurt
- 1 garlic clove, diced

1. Put all ingredients in the blender and blend until smooth.
2. Transfer the spread in the serving bowl.

per serving: 229 calories, 3.8g protein, 11.3g carbohydrates, 20g fat, 6.8g fiber, 0mg cholesterol, 28mg sodium, 565mg potassium

Burrito Bowl

Prep time: 10 minutes | **Cook time:** 0 minutes | **Servings:** 4

- 4 tomatoes, chopped
- 1 cucumber, chopped
- ¼ cup quinoa, cooked
- 2 tablespoons plain
- yogurt
- 1 teaspoon ground coriander
- 1 teaspoon chili powder
- ¼ cup fresh cilantro, chopped

1. Put all ingredients in the serving bowls and carefully mix them.

per serving: 81 calories, 3.7g protein, 15.4g carbohydrates, 1.2g fat, 2.9g fiber, 0mg cholesterol, 21mg sodium, 511mg potassium

Grilled Peppers

Prep time: 10 minutes | **Cook time:** 8 minutes | **Servings:** 4

- 4 sweet peppers
- 1 tablespoon olive oil
- 1 teaspoon fresh
- parsley, chopped
- 1 teaspoon sesame seeds

1. Preheat the grill to 400F.
2. Put the sweet peppers in the grill and cook for 4 minutes per side.
3. Then peel the sweet peppers and chop them roughly.
4. Mix the chopped peppers with olive oil, parsley, and sesame seeds.

per serving: 72 calories, 1.3g protein, 9.2g carbohydrates, 4.2g fat, 1.7g fiber, 0mg cholesterol, 3mg sodium, 229mg potassium

Parsley Guacamole

Prep time: 10 minutes | **Cook time:** 0 minutes | **Servings:** 4

- 1 avocado, pitted, peeled and chopped
- ½ cup chopped parsley
- 2 lemons
- ¼ cup coconut cream

1. Mix avocado with parsley and coconut cream.
2. Gently blend the mixture.
3. Then squeeze the lemon juice in the avocado mixture.
4. Carefully mix the meal.

per serving: 148 calories, 1.8g protein, 8.3g carbohydrates, 13.5g fat, 4.8g fiber, 0mg cholesterol, 10mg sodium, 365mg potassium

Baked Celery Root

Prep time: 10 minutes | **Cook time:** 35 minutes | **Servings:** 4

- 12 oz celery root, peeled, roughly chopped
- 1 teaspoon ground coriander
- 1 tablespoon olive oil

1. Mix celery root with ground coriander and olive oil.
2. Put the vegetable in the baking tray and bake at 365F for 30 minutes.

per serving: 66 calories, 1.3g protein, 7.8g carbohydrates, 3.8g fat, 1.5g fiber, 0mg cholesterol, 85mg sodium, 256mg potassium

Baked Chickpeas

Prep time: 10 minutes | **Cook time:** 20 minutes | **Servings:** 4

- 2 cups chickpeas, boiled
- 1 tablespoon olive oil
- 1 teaspoon chili powder
- 1 teaspoon ground black pepper
- 1 tablespoon dried oregano

1. Line the baking tray with baking paper.
2. Then mix chickpeas with olive oil, chili powder, ground black pepper, and dried oregano.
3. Put the mixture in the baking tray and bake at 365F for 20 minutes.

per serving: 401 calories, 19.6g protein, 62.1g carbohydrates, 9.8g fat, 18.2g fiber, 0mg cholesterol, 31mg sodium, 913mg potassium

Turmeric Swiss Chard

Prep time: 25 minutes | **Cook time:** 0 minutes | **Servings:** 4

- 1-pound swiss chard, chopped
- 3 oz tofu, cubed
- 1 teaspoon ground turmeric
- 2 tablespoons lemon juice
- 1 teaspoon lemon zest, grated
- 1 teaspoon minced ginger
- 1 tablespoon olive oil

1. In the mixing bowl, mix ground turmeric with lemon juice, lemon zest, minced ginger, and olive oil.
2. Add tofu and mix the mixture well. Leave tofu for 10 minutes.
3. Then mix tofu mixture with swiss chard.

per serving: 73 calories, 3.9g protein, 5.5g carbohydrates, 4.8g fat, 2.3g fiber, 0mg cholesterol, 247mg sodium, 493mg potassium

Cheese and Green Peas Casserole

Prep time: 10 minutes | **Cook time:** 30 minutes | **Servings:** 6

- 2 cups green peas, frozen
- ¼ cup of coconut milk
- 5 oz Romano cheese, grated
- 1 teaspoon olive oil

1. Brush the casserole mold with olive oil from inside.
2. Then mix green peas with coconut milk and pour the mixture in the casserole mold. Flatten it well and sprinkle with Romano cheese.
3. Bake the casserole for 30 minutes at 355F.

per serving: 160 calories, 10.4g protein, 8.4g carbohydrates, 9.7g fat, 2.7g fiber, 25mg cholesterol, 287mg sodium, 165mg potassium

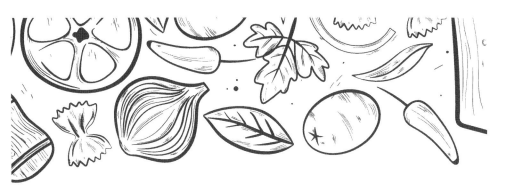

Sauces, Condiments & Dressings

Basil Dressing

Prep time: 10 minutes | **Cook time:** 0 minutes | **Servings:** 4

- ½ cup fresh basil
- 4 tablespoons lemon juice
- 1 tablespoon olive oil

1. Blend the basil until smooth.
2. Then mix it with lemon juice and olive oil.

per serving: 34 calories, 0.2g protein, 0.4g carbohydrates, 3.6g fat, 0.1g fiber, 0mg cholesterol, 3mg sodium, 28mg potassium.

Garlic Confit

Prep time: 10 minutes | **Cook time:** 20 minutes | **Servings:** 4

- 6 oz garlic cloves, peeled
- ¼ cup of water
- ¼ cup apple cider vinegar
- 1 teaspoon dried basil
- ½ teaspoon peppercorns

1. Pour water in the saucepan.
2. Bring it to boil.
3. Add garlic cloves and all remaining ingredients.
4. Transfer the mixture in the glass jar and close the lid.

per serving: 67 calories, 2.7g protein, 14.4g carbohydrates, 0.2g fat, 1g fiber, 0mg cholesterol, 9mg sodium, 186mg potassium.

Hot Dressing

Prep time: 10 minutes | **Cook time:** 0 minutes | **Servings:** 4

5 jalapenos, minced
- 3 tablespoons fresh parsley, chopped
- 1 tablespoon
- minced garlic
- 3 tablespoons olive oil

1. Put all ingredients in the blender and blend until smooth.

per serving: 99 calories, 0.5g protein, 1.9g carbohydrates, 10.6g fat, 0.6g fiber, 0mg cholesterol, 2mg sodium, 62mg potassium.

Strawberry Sauce

Prep time: 10 minutes | **Cook time:** 0 minutes | **Servings:** 4

- 1 cup strawberries
- 3 tablespoons olive oil
- 1 tablespoon apple cider vinegar

1. Blend the strawberries until smooth.
2. Then mix the strawberry mixture with olive oil and apple cider vinegar.

per serving: 102 calories, 0.2g protein, 2.8g carbohydrates, 10.6g fat, 0.7g fiber, 0mg cholesterol, 1mg sodium, 58mg potassium.

Chipotle Sauce

Prep time: 10 minutes | **Cook time:** 0 minutes | **Servings:** 4

- 2 chipotles, blended
- 2 tablespoons plain yogurt
- 1 teaspoon dried cilantro
- 1 tablespoon balsamic vinegar

1. In the mixing bowl, mix chipotles with plain yogurt, dried cilantro, and balsamic vinegar.
2. Carefully mix the sauce.

per serving: 6 calories, 0.4g protein, 0.6g carbohydrates, 0.1g fat, 0g fiber, 0mg cholesterol, 6mg sodium, 21mg potassium.

Hot Ketchup

Prep time: 10 minutes | **Cook time:** 15 minutes | **Servings:** 4

- 2 cups tomatoes, chopped
- 1 teaspoon dried basil
- 1 jalapeno pepper, minced
- 1 teaspoon minced garlic
- 1 chili pepper, minced

1. Blend the tomatoes until smooth and pour them in the saucepan.
2. Add dried basil, jalapeno pepper, garlic, and chili pepper.
3. Bring the ketchup to boil.

per serving: 19 calories, 0.9g protein, 4g carbohydrates, 0.2g fat, 1.2g fiber, 0mg cholesterol, 5mg sodium, 227mg potassium.

Curry Dressing

Prep time: 10 minutes | **Cook time:** 0 minutes | **Servings:** 4

- 1 tablespoon tahini paste
- 2 tablespoons lemon juice
- 1 teaspoon curry paste
- 1 teaspoon olive oil

1. Mix curry paste with lemon juice.
2. Then add tahini paste and olive oil.

per serving: 43 calories, 0.8g protein, 1.3g carbohydrates, 4g fat, 0.4g fiber, 0mg cholesterol, 6mg sodium, 25mg potassium.

Lemon Pepper Dressing

Prep time: 10 minutes | **Cook time:** 0 minutes | **Servings:** 4

- 1 teaspoon lemon pepper seasonings
- 3 tablespoons apple cider vinegar
- 1 tablespoon olive oil
- 2 tablespoons orange juice

1. Mix lemon pepper seasonings with apple cider vinegar.
2. Add olive oil and orange juice.
3. Whisk the dressing.

per serving: 37 calories, 0.1g protein, 1.3g carbohydrates, 3.5g fat, 0.2g fiber, 0mg cholesterol, 1mg sodium, 30mg potassium.

Berries BBQ Sauce

Prep time: 10 minutes | **Cook time:** 0 minutes | **Servings:** 4

- 1 cup blueberries
- 2 tablespoons apple cider
- vinegar
- 1 tablespoon raw honey

1. Blend the blueberries until you get a smooth mixture.
2. Add apple cider vinegar and raw honey.
3. Whisk the mixture well.

per serving: 38 calories, 0.3g protein, 9.7g carbohydrates, 0.1g fat, 0.9g fiber, 0mg cholesterol, 1mg sodium, 36mg potassium.

Sweet Dressing

Prep time: 10 minutes | **Cook time:** 0 minutes | **Servings:** 4

- 2 tablespoons raw honey
- 2 tablespoons Dijon mustard

1. In the shallow bowl whisk raw honey with Mustard.

per serving: 37 calories, 0.4g protein, 9.1g carbohydrates, 0.3g fat, 0.3g fiber, 0mg cholesterol, 89mg sodium, 16mg potassium.

Peanut Dressing

Prep time: 10 minutes | **Cook time:** 0 minutes | **Servings:** 4

- 1 tablespoon tahini paste
- 2 tablespoons
- peanut butter
- 1 tablespoon lemon juice

1. Whisk all ingredients in the shallow bowl.

per serving: 70 calories, 2.7g protein, 2.5g carbohydrates, 6.1g fat, 0.9g fiber, 0mg cholesterol, 42mg sodium, 72mg potassium.

Balsamic Dressing

Prep time: 10 minutes | **Cook time:** 0 minutes | **Servings:** 4

- 1 tablespoon minced garlic
- 5 tablespoons
- balsamic vinegar
- 2 tablespoons olive oil

1. Mix all ingredients in the bowl.
2. Whisk gently.

per serving: 67 calories, 0.1g protein, 0.9g carbohydrates, 7g fat, 0g fiber, 0mg cholesterol, 1mg sodium, 22mg potassium.

Low-Fat Mayo

Prep time: 10 minutes | **Cook time:** 0 minutes | **Servings:** 4

- 2 tablespoons mustard
- ½ cup olive oil
- 1 egg, beaten
- 1 tablespoon lemon juice

1. Put all ingredients in the blender,
2. Blend the mixture until it is smooth.

per serving: 259 calories, 2.8g protein, 2.1g carbohydrates, 27.9g fat, 0.8g fiber, 41mg cholesterol, 16mg sodium, 58mg potassium.

Garlic Dressing

Prep time: 10 minutes | **Cook time:** 0 minutes | **Servings:** 4

- 1 teaspoon minced garlic
- 2 tablespoons
- balsamic vinegar
- 1 tablespoon olive oil

1. Mix minced garlic with balsamic vinegar and olive oil.
2. Whisk the mixture.

per serving: 33 calories, 0g protein, 0.3g carbohydrates, 3.5g fat, 0g fiber, 0mg cholesterol, 1mg sodium, 8mg potassium.

Hot Strawberry Sauce

Prep time: 10 minutes | **Cook time:** 10 minutes | **Servings:** 4

- 2 jalapenos, chopped
- ½ cup strawberries, chopped
- 1 onion, chopped
- 1 teaspoon orange zest, grated
- 1 tablespoon avocado oil

1. Put all ingredients in the blender and blend until smooth.
2. Then pour the mixture in the saucepan and bring it to boil.
3. Cool the sauce to the room temperature.

per serving: 24 calories, 0.6g protein, 4.7g carbohydrates, 0.6g fat, 1.4g fiber, 0mg cholesterol, 2mg sodium, 95mg potassium.

Sweet and Sauer Sauce

Prep time: 10 minutes | **Cook time:** 20 minutes | **Servings:** 4

- ¼ cup lemon juice
- 1 tablespoon liquid honey
- 1 teaspoon chili
- flakes
- 1 tablespoon olive oil

1. Mix lemon juice with liquid honey.
2. Add chili flakes and olive oil.
3. Stir the sauce.

per serving: 50 calories, 0.2g protein, 4.7g carbohydrates, 3.6g fat, 0.1g fiber, 0mg cholesterol, 3mg sodium, 23mg potassium.

Pesto Sauce

Prep time: 10 minutes | **Cook time:** 0 minutes | **Servings:** 8

- 1 oz parmesan, grated
- 1 cup basil, chopped
- 1 oz pinenuts
- 1 teaspoon ground black pepper
- 1/3 cup olive oil

1. Blend basil with pinenuts, ground black pepper, and olive oil.
2. When the mixture is smooth, add Parmesan.
3. Stir the sauce.

per serving: 109 calories, 1.8g protein, 1.5g carbohydrates, 11.1g fat, 0.6g fiber, 3mg cholesterol, 33mg sodium, 12mg potassium.

Lime Dressing

Prep time: 10 minutes | **Cook time:** 0 minutes | **Servings:** 4

- ½ cup lime juice
- 1 cup fresh cilantro, chopped
- ¼ teaspoon
- ground nutmeg
- 1 tablespoon olive oil

1. Mix lime juice with fresh cilantro, ground nutmeg, and olive oil.
2. Whisk the dressing.

per serving: 38 calories, 0.2g protein, 2.3g carbohydrates, 3.6g fat, 0.3g fiber, 0mg cholesterol, 7mg sodium, 44mg potassium.

Fast Salad Dressing

Prep time: 10 minutes | **Cook time:** 0 minutes | **Servings:** 4

- ¼ cup of orange juice
- 1 tablespoon Dijon mustard
- 1 teaspoon raw
- honey
- 1 tablespoon apple cider vinegar
- 1 teaspoon dried basil

1. Whisk all ingredients in the bowl until you get a homogenous mixture.

per serving: 16 calories, 0.3g protein, 3.3g carbohydrates, 0.2g fat, 0.2g fiber, 0mg cholesterol, 45mg sodium, 41mg potassium.

Basil Vinaigrette

Prep time: 10 minutes | **Cook time:** 20 minutes | **Servings:** 4

- ¼ cup lemon juice
- ¼ cup fresh basil, blended
- 1 tablespoon raw honey

1. Mix lemon juice with raw honey.
2. When the liquid is smooth, add fresh basil and stir well.

per serving: 20 calories, 0.2g protein, 4.7g carbohydrates, 0.1g fat, 0.1g fiber, 4.7mg cholesterol, 3mg sodium, 26mg potassium.

Creamy Dressing

Prep time: 10 minutes | **Cook time:** 0 minutes | **Servings:** 4

- 1 avocado, pitted, peeled
- ¼ cup coconut cream
- ¼ cup lemon juice
- ½ teaspoon ground coriander

1. Blend the avocado until smooth.
2. Then add coconut cream, lemon juice, and ground coriander.
3. Stir the mixture well.

per serving: 141 calories, 1.4g protein, 5.5g carbohydrates, 13.5g fat, 3.8g fiber, 0mg cholesterol, 8mg sodium, 302mg potassium.

Cashew Sauce

Prep time: 10 minutes | **Cook time:** 0 minutes | **Servings:** 4

- ½ cup cashew
- ¼ cup lemon juice
- ¼ water
- 1 teaspoon ground
- black pepper
- ¼ cup fresh cilantro

1. Blend the cashews with water and lemon juice.
2. Add ground black pepper and fresh cilantro.
3. Blend the sauce until smooth.

per serving: 104 calories, 2.8g protein, 6.3g carbohydrates, 8.1g fat, 0.7g fiber, 0mg cholesterol, 7mg sodium, 128mg potassium.

Chili Pepper Sauce

Prep time: 10 minutes | **Cook time:** 0 minutes | **Servings:** 4

- 1 tomato, chopped
- 3 chilies
- 1 tablespoon fresh parsley
- 1 tablespoon olive oil
- 1 teaspoon lime juice

1. Put all ingredients in the blender.
2. Blend the mixture until you get a smooth sauce.

per serving: 35 calories, 0.2g protein, 1.1g carbohydrates, 3.6g fat, 0.3g fiber, 0mg cholesterol, 2mg sodium, 51mg potassium.

Onion Dressing

Prep time: 10 minutes | **Cook time:** 0 minutes | **Servings:** 4

- 1 red onion, minced
- 3 tablespoons olive oil
- 2 tablespoons lemon juice
- 1 teaspoon chili flakes

1. Mix onion with olive oil.
2. Then add lemon juice and chili flakes. Stir the dressing.

per serving: 24 calories, 0.6g protein, 4.7g carbohydrates, 0.6g fat, 1.4g fiber, 0mg cholesterol, 2mg sodium, 95mg potassium.

Chimichurri Sauce

Prep time: 10 minutes | **Cook time:** 0 minutes | **Servings:** 4

- ½ cup cilantro
- 1 tablespoon garlic
- 2 jalapenos, chopped
- 2 oz parsley, chopped
- 3 tablespoons apple cider vinegar
- 5 tablespoons olive oil

1. Put all ingredients in the blender.
2. Blend the sauce until smooth.

per serving: 163 calories, 0.7g protein, 2.2g carbohydrates, 17.7g fat, 0.8g fiber, 0mg cholesterol, 10mg sodium, 121mg potassium.

Toasted Almonds Sauce

Prep time: 10 minutes | **Cook time:** 0 minutes | **Servings:** 4

- ¼ cup almonds, toasted, grinded
- 1 avocado, chopped
- ¼ cup coconut cream
- 1 teaspoon chili powder

1. Blend the avocado until smooth.
2. Then mix blended avocado with almonds, coconut cream, and chili powder.

per serving: 173 calories, 2.6g protein, 6.8g carbohydrates, 16.5g fat, 4.7g fiber, 0mg cholesterol, 12mg sodium, 339mg potassium.

Horseradish Sauce

Prep time: 10 minutes | **Cook time:** 0 minutes | **Servings:** 4

- 6 oz horseradish, grated
- 2 oz beet, peeled, grated
- 4 tablespoons apple cider vinegar

1. Mix horseradish with beet and apple cider vinegar.
2. Stir the sauce well.

per serving: 30 calories, 0.7g protein, 6.4g carbohydrates, 0.3g fat, 1.7g fiber, 0mg cholesterol, 145mg sodium, 159mg potassium.

Ginger Dressing

Prep time: 10 minutes | **Cook time:** 0 minutes | **Servings:** 4

- 1 tablespoon minced ginger
- 1 tablespoon olive oil
- 1 teaspoon dried dill

1. Whisk the minced ginger with olive oil.
2. Add dried dill, carefully mix the dressing.

per serving: 35 calories, 0.2g protein, 1.1g carbohydrates, 3.6g fat, 0.2g fiber, 0mg cholesterol, 1mg sodium, 26mg potassium.

Mango Sauce

Prep time: 10 minutes | **Cook time:** 0 minutes | **Servings:** 4

- 1 mango, pitted, peeled, chopped
- 2 tablespoons lemon juice
- 1 teaspoon ground paprika
- 1 tablespoon olive oil

1. Blend the mango until smooth.
2. Add lemon juice, ground paprika, and olive oil.
3. Stir the sauce.

per serving: 84 calories, 0.8g protein, 13g carbohydrates, 4g fat, 1.6g fiber, 0mg cholesterol, 3mg sodium, 163mg potassium.

Mint Dressing

Prep time: 10 minutes | **Cook time:** 0 minutes | **Servings:** 4

- 1 tablespoon mustard
- 1 teaspoon fresh mint, grinded
- 2 tablespoons olive oil
- 4 tablespoons orange juice

1. Put all ingredients in the blender.
2. Blend the dressing until smooth.

per serving: 80 calories, 0.8g protein, 2.6g carbohydrates, 7.8g fat, 0.5g fiber, 0mg cholesterol, 0mg sodium, 52mg potassium.

Herbs Vinaigrette

Prep time: 10 minutes | **Cook time:** 0 minutes | **Servings:** 4

- 1 teaspoon cumin seeds
- ¼ teaspoon coriander seeds
- ¼ teaspoon fennel seeds
- 1 teaspoon dried lemongrass
- 5 tablespoons olive oil
- 3 tablespoons lemon juice

1. Put all ingredients in the glass jar.
2. Shake the vinaigrette well.

per serving: 156 calories, 0.2g protein, 0.6g carbohydrates, 17.7g fat, 0.2g fiber, 0mg cholesterol, 0mg sodium, 29mg potassium.

Pomegranate Dressing

Prep time: 10 minutes | **Cook time:** 0 minutes | **Servings:** 4

- ¼ cup pomegranate juice
- ½ teaspoon lemon zest, grated
- ¼ teaspoon ground turmeric
- ¼ teaspoon minced ginger

1. Mix pomegranate juice with lemon zest and ground turmeric.
2. Add minced ginger.

per serving: 10 calories, 0g protein, 2.5g carbohydrates, 0g fat, 0.1g fiber, 0mg cholesterol, 1mg sodium, 43mg potassium.

Cucumber Sauce

Prep time: 10 minutes | **Cook time:** 0 minutes | **Servings:** 4

- 1 cucumber, grated
- 1 oz chives, chopped
- ¼ cup plain yogurt
- 1 teaspoon ground black pepper

1. Mix cucumber with chives, plain yogurt, and ground black pepper.
2. Stir the sauce well.

per serving: 26 calories, 1.7g protein, 4.5g carbohydrates, 0.3g fat, 0.7g fiber, 1mg cholesterol, 13mg sodium, 174mg potassium.

Sweet Pepper Paste

Prep time: 10 minutes | **Cook time:** 10 minutes | **Servings:** 4

- 2 cups sweet peppers, chopped
- 3 tablespoons olive oil
- 1 teaspoon ground cumin

1. Grill the peppers for 4 minutes per side at 400F.
2. Then peel the peppers and put them in the blender.
3. Add all remaining ingredients and blend until smooth.

per serving: 111 calories, 0.7g protein, 4.7g carbohydrates, 10.8g fat, 0.9g fiber, 0mg cholesterol, 2mg sodium, 121mg potassium.

Apples Salad Dressing

Prep time: 10 minutes | **Cook time:** 0 minutes | **Servings:** 4

- ½ teaspoon dried thyme
- ½ teaspoon dried oregano
- 2 tablespoons olive oil
- ¼ cup apple juice
- ¼ teaspoon dried rosemary

1. Put all ingredients in the glass jar.
2. Shake the dressing well.

per serving: 68 calories, 0g protein, 2g carbohydrates, 7.1g fat, 0.2g fiber, 0mg cholesterol, 1mg sodium, 21mg potassium.

Avocado Ranch Dressing

Prep time: 10 minutes | **Cook time:** 0 minutes | **Servings:** 4

- ½ cup fresh dill, chopped
- 1 avocado, pitted, peeled, chopped
- 2 garlic cloves, peeled
- 4 tablespoons olive oil
- 1 teaspoon chili powder

1. Put all ingredients in the food processor.
2. Blend the mixture until smooth.

per serving: 242 calories, 2.3g protein, 8.5g carbohydrates, 24.2g fat, 8.8g fiber, 0mg cholesterol, 22mg sodium, 461mg potassium.

Olives Dressing

Prep time: 10 minutes | **Cook time:** 0 minutes | **Servings:** 4

- 4 tablespoons olive oil
- ¼ cup Olives, blended
- 1 teaspoon dried rosemary
- 3 tablespoons lime juice

1. Mix olives with olive oil, dried rosemary, and lime juice.
2. Stir the dressing gently.

per serving: 132 calories, 0.1g protein, 1.2g carbohydrates, 15g fat, 0.4g fiber, 0mg cholesterol, 75mg sodium, 9mg potassium.

Tahini Dressing

Prep time: 10 minutes | **Cook time:** 0 minutes | **Servings:** 4

- 1 tablespoon tahini paste
- 1 teaspoon liquid honey
- 1 teaspoon lemon juice
- 1 teaspoon ground turmeric

1. Mix tahini paste with liquid honey.
2. Add lemon juice and ground turmeric.
3. Stir the dressing.

per serving: 30 calories, 0.7g protein, 2.6g carbohydrates, 2.1g fat, 0.5g fiber, 0mg cholesterol, 5mg sodium, 32mg potassium.

Balsamic Vinaigrette

Prep time: 10 minutes | **Cook time:** 0 minutes | **Servings:** 8

- 3 tablespoons balsamic vinegar
- 1 teaspoon mustard
- 1 teaspoon minced garlic
- 6 tablespoons olive oil

1. Mix balsamic vinegar with mustard, minced garlic, and olive oil.
2. Whisk the mixture well.

per serving: 94 calories, 0.1g protein, 0.3g carbohydrates, 10.6g fat, 0.1g fiber, 0mg cholesterol, 0mg sodium, 8mg potassium.

Anti-Inflammatory Oil

Prep time: 10 minutes | **Cook time:** 0 minutes | **Servings:** 4

- ¼ cup olive oil
- 1 tablespoon dried thyme
- 2 tablespoons
- dried rosemary
- 1 garlic clove, peeled

1. Put all ingredients in the can and close the lid.
2. Leave the oil for 1-2 days in the fridge.

per serving: 116 calories, 0.2g protein, 1.7g carbohydrates, 12.9g fat, 1g fiber, 0mg cholesterol, 1mg sodium, 24mg potassium.

Mustard Dressing

Prep time: 10 minutes | **Cook time:** 0 minutes | **Servings:** 4

- 1 egg, beaten
- 3 tablespoons mustard
- 3 tablespoons lemon juice

1. Whisk the egg.
2. Then add mustard and lemon juice.
3. Stir the dressing.

per serving: 58 calories, 3.6g protein, 3.3g carbohydrates, 3.6g fat, 1.3g fiber, 41mg cholesterol, 18mg sodium, 86mg potassium.

Honey Sauce

Prep time: 10 minutes | **Cook time:** 0 minutes | **Servings:** 4

- 2 tablespoons of liquid honey
- ¼ cup of orange juice
- 1 teaspoon ground cinnamon
- ½ teaspoon chili flakes

1. Put all ingredients in the blender,
2. Blend the sauce until smooth.

per serving: 40 calories, 0.2g protein, 10.7g carbohydrates, 0g fat, 0.4g fiber, 0mg cholesterol, 1mg sodium, 40mg potassium.

Turmeric Dressing

Prep time: 10 minutes | **Cook time:** 0 minutes | **Servings:** 4

- 1 tablespoon ground turmeric
- 1 teaspoon minced ginger
- 1 teaspoon minced
- garlic
- 3 tablespoons coconut cream
- 1 tablespoon liquid honey

1. Put all ingredients in the blender.
2. Blend the dressing until smooth.

per serving: 50 calories, 0.5g protein, 6.6g carbohydrates, 2.9g fat, 0.7g fiber, 0mg cholesterol, 3mg sodium, 84mg potassium.

Spinach Dressing

Prep time: 10 minutes | **Cook time:** 0 minutes | **Servings:** 4

- 1 cup spinach, blended
- 3 tablespoons olive
- oil
- 3 tablespoons lemon juice

1. Whisk the spinach with olive oil.
2. Add lemon juice and stir the dressing.

per serving: 94 calories, 0.3g protein, 0.5g carbohydrates, 10.6g fat, 0.2g fiber, 0mg cholesterol, 8mg sodium, 56mg potassium.

Peanut Dressing

Prep time: 10 minutes | Cook time: 0 minutes | Servings: 4

- 2 tablespoons peanut butter
- 1 tablespoon plain
- yogurt
- ½ teaspoon mustard seeds

1. Mix peanut butter with mustard seeds.
2. Add plain yogurt.
3. Stir the dressing.

per serving: 52 calories, 2.3g protein, 2g carbohydrates, 4.2g fat, 0.5g fiber, 0mg cholesterol, 39mg sodium, 64mg potassium.

Avocado Condiment

Prep time: 10 minutes | Cook time: 0 minutes | Servings: 4

- 1 avocado, pitted, peeled
- 2 tablespoons lemon juice
- ¼ cup fresh cilantro, chopped
- 1 jalapeno, chopped

1. Dice the avocado and mix it with lemon juice, cilantro, and jalapeno pepper.
2. Stir the mixture.

per serving: 106 calories, 1.1g protein, 4.7g carbohydrates, 9.9g fat, 3.5g fiber, 0mg cholesterol, 5mg sodium, 266mg potassium.

Almond Sauce

Prep time: 10 minutes | Cook time: 0 minutes | Servings: 4

- 1 avocado, pitted, peeled, chopped
- ¼ cup almonds
- ¼ cup of coconut milk

1. Put all ingredients in the blender.
2. Blend the sauce until smooth.

per serving: 171 calories, 2.6g protein, 6.4g carbohydrates, 16.4g fat, 4.4g fiber, 0mg cholesterol, 5mg sodium, 327mg potassium.

Tomato Sauce

Prep time: 10 minutes | Cook time: 10 minutes | Servings: 4

- 1 cup tomatoes, chopped
- 1 teaspoon dried rosemary
- ½ teaspoon garlic, minced
- ½ teaspoon dried basil

1. Blend the tomatoes until smooth and pour the mixture in the saucepan.
2. Add all remaining ingredients and bring the sauce to boil.

per serving: 10 calories, 0.4g protein, 2.1g carbohydrates, 0.1g fat, 0.7g fiber, 0mg cholesterol, 2mg sodium, 111mg potassium.

Greek-Style Dressing

Prep time: 10 minutes | Cook time: 0 minutes | Servings: 4

- ½ cup plain yogurt
- 1 tablespoon Italian seasonings

1. Put plain yogurt and Italian seasonings in the bowl and stir well.

per serving: 33 calories, 1.8g protein, 2.5g carbohydrates, 1.4g fat, 0g fiber, 4mg cholesterol, 23mg sodium, 73mg potassium.

Avocado Sauce

Prep time: 10 minutes | Cook time: 0 minutes | Servings: 4

- 3 tablespoons coconut cream
- 1 avocado, pitted,
- peeled, chopped
- ½ cup fresh dill

1. Put the avocado in the blender and blend until smooth.
2. Add dill and coconut cream and blend the mixture for 1 minute more.

per serving: 144 calories, 2.4g protein, 8.3g carbohydrates, 12.7g fat, 4.4g fiber, 0mg cholesterol, 17mg sodium, 472mg potassium.

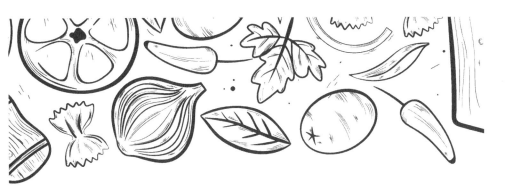

Smoothies & Drinks

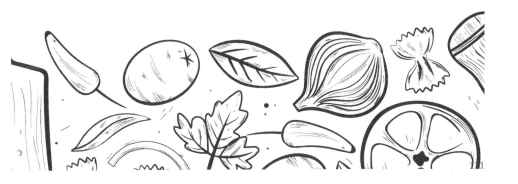

Pineapple Smoothie

Prep time: 10 minutes | **Cook time:** 0 minutes | **Servings:** 1

- 1 cup pineapple, chopped
- ¼ cup of coconut milk

1. Put pineapple in the blender and blend until smooth.
2. Then add coconut milk and blend the mixture until homogenous.

per serving: 220 calories, 2.3g protein, 25g carbohydrates, 14.5g fat, 3.6g fiber, 0mg cholesterol, 11mg sodium, 338mg potassium.

Zucchini Smoothie

Prep time: 10 minutes | **Cook time:** 0 minutes | **Servings:** 2

- 2 cups zucchini, chopped
- 1 teaspoon ground paprika
- 1 cup of water

1. Blend the zucchini until smooth.
2. Then add water and ground paprika.
3. Pulse the smoothies for 10 seconds.

per serving: 21 calories, 1.5g protein, 4.4g carbohydrates, 0.3g fat, 1.6g fiber, 0mg cholesterol, 15mg sodium, 322mg potassium.

Mango and Cherries Smoothie

Prep time: 5 minutes | **Cook time:** 0 minutes | **Servings:** 4

- 1 cup cherries, pitted
- 1 teaspoon dried mint
- 1 mango, peeled, chopped
- 1 orange, peeled, chopped
- 1 cup of water

1. Put all ingredients in the blender.
2. Blend the smoothie until it is smooth and pour in the glasses.

per serving: 87 calories, 1.4g protein, 21.5g carbohydrates, 0.4g fat, 3g fiber, 0mg cholesterol, 5mg sodium, 227mg potassium.

Raspberry Smoothie

Prep time: 10 minutes | **Cook time:** 0 minutes | **Servings:** 2

- 2 oranges, peeled, chopped
- ½ cup of water
- ½ cup raspberries

1. Blend the raspberries with oranges until smooth.
2. Then add water and blend the mixture for 5 seconds more.

per serving: 102 calories, 2.1g protein, 25.3g carbohydrates, 0.4g fat, 6.4g fiber, 0mg cholesterol, 2mg sodium, 380mg potassium.

Mint and Beet Smoothie

Prep time: 10 minutes | **Cook time:** 0 minutes | **Servings:** 2

- 2 cups beets, chopped
- mint
- 1 cup of water
- 1 tablespoon fresh

1. Put all ingredients in the blender and blend until smooth.

per serving: 76 calories, 3g protein, 17.2g carbohydrates, 0.3g fat, 3.6g fiber, 0mg cholesterol, 135mg sodium, 533mg potassium.

Light Smoothie

Prep time: 5 minutes | **Cook time:** 0 minutes | **Servings:** 2

- 2 cups raspberries
- ½ cup of coconut milk

1. Blend raspberries with coconut milk until smooth.

per serving: 202 calories, 2.9g protein, 18g carbohydrates, 15.1g fat, 9.3g fiber, 0mg cholesterol, 10mg sodium, 344mg potassium.

Sweet Kale Smoothie

Prep time: 5 minutes | **Cook time:** 0 minutes | **Servings:** 4

- 1 cup kale, chopped
- ½ cup of coconut milk
- 3 cups grapes, chopped
- 1 oz pistachios, chopped

1. Blend all ingredients in the blender.
2. Pour the smoothies in the serving glasses.

per serving: 161 calories, 3g protein, 17.1g carbohydrates, 10.7g fat, 2.2g fiber, 0mg cholesterol, 51mg sodium, 366mg potassium.

Pink Smoothie

Prep time: 5 minutes | **Cook time:** 0 minutes | **Servings:** 2

- 1 banana, chopped
- 1 cup cherries,
- pitted
- ½ cup of water

1. Mix banana with cherries until smooth.
2. Then add water and mix well.

per serving: 83 calories, 1.1g protein, 20.5g carbohydrates, 0.2g fat, 2.5g fiber, 0mg cholesterol, 7mg sodium, 212mg potassium.

Blackberries Smoothie

Prep time: 10 minutes | **Cook time:** 0 minutes | **Servings:** 2

- 1 cup blackberries
- 1 cup parsley, chopped
- ½ cup of coconut milk

1. Blend all ingredients in the blender until smooth.
2. Serve the cooked smoothie with ice cubes.

per serving: 180 calories, 3.3g protein, 12.1g carbohydrates, 14.9g fat, 6.1g fiber, 0mg cholesterol, 27mg sodium, 441mg potassium.

Nutmeg Smoothie

Prep time: 5 minutes | **Cook time:** 0 minutes | **Servings:** 2

- 1 teaspoon ground nutmeg
- 2 mangos, peeled,
- chopped
- ½ cup of coconut milk

1. Mix mangos with coconut milk and blend until smooth.
2. Pour the smoothie in the glasses and top with ground nutmeg.

per serving: 345 calories, 4.2g protein, 54.2g carbohydrates, 16g fat, 6.9g fiber, 0mg cholesterol, 13mg sodium, 726mg potassium.

Ginger Tea

Prep time: 15 minutes | **Cook time:** 15 minutes | **Servings:** 4

- 2 tablespoons ground ginger
- ½ lemon
- 5 cups of water
- 1 oz cranberries
- 1 tablespoon liquid honey

1. Bring the water to boil.
2. Add cranberries, ground ginger, and juice from ½ of lemon.
3. Simmer the tea for 5 minutes.
4. Then add honey.

per serving: 31 calories, 0.4g protein, 7.6g carbohydrates, 0.2g fat, 0.8g fiber, 0mg cholesterol, 10mg sodium, 64mg potassium.

Greens Smoothie

Prep time: 5 minutes | **Cook time:** 0 minutes | **Servings:** 4

- 1 cup arugula, chopped
- 1 cup spinach, chopped
- 1 cup lettuce, chopped
- 1 cup of water
- 1 teaspoon salt

1. Put all ingredients from the list above in the blender.
2. Blend the smoothie until smooth.

per serving: 5 calories, 0.4g protein, 0.9g carbohydrates, 0.1g fat, 0.3g fiber, 0mg cholesterol, 591mg sodium, 80mg potassium.

Cinnamon and Blueberries Smoothie

Prep time: 5 minutes | **Cook time:** 0 minutes | **Servings:** 4

- 1 teaspoon ground cinnamon
- 2 cups blueberries
- 2 cups of coconut milk

1. Mix blueberries with coconut milk and blend until smooth.
2. Add ground cinnamon and pour in the serving glasses.

per serving: 319 calories, 3.3g protein, 17.6g carbohydrates, 28.9g fat, 4.7g fiber, 0mg cholesterol, 19mg sodium, 374mg potassium.

Coconut Smoothie

Prep time: 5 minutes | **Cook time:** 0 minutes | **Servings:** 4

- 2 cups of coconut milk
- 3 oz coconut shred
- 2 oz almonds,
- chopped
- 1 tablespoon liquid honey

1. Grind almonds and mix them with coconut milk, coconut shred, and liquid honey.
2. Stir the smoothie and pour in the glasses.

per serving: 480 calories, 6.4g protein, 24.2g carbohydrates, 43.3g fat, 5.4g fiber, 0mg cholesterol, 74mg sodium, 494mg potassium.

Pears Smoothie

Prep time: 5 minutes | **Cook time:** 0 minutes | **Servings:** 4

- 2 cups pears, chopped
- 1 avocado,
- chopped
- 1 cup of water

1. Blend the avocado with pears.
2. When the mixture is smooth, add water and gently mix.

per serving: 149 calories, 1.2g protein, 16.6g carbohydrates, 9.9g fat, 5.9g fiber, 0mg cholesterol, 6mg sodium, 338mg potassium.

Pepper Smoothie

Prep time: 5 minutes | **Cook time:** 0 minutes | **Servings:** 4

- 2 cups peppers, chopped
- 1 cup of water
- 1 cup arugula, chopped
- ½ cup lettuce, chopped
- 1 teaspoon chili powder

1. Blend all ingredients in the blender.
2. When the smoothies are smooth, pour it in the glasses.

per serving: 53 calories, 2.3g protein, 13.2g carbohydrates, 0.8g fat, 5.4g fiber, 0mg cholesterol, 19mg sodium, 283mg potassium.

Spinach and Radish Smoothie

Prep time: 5 minutes | **Cook time:** 0 minutes | **Servings:** 4

- 1 cup radish, chopped
- 2 cups spinach, chopped
- 1 cup of coconut
- milk
- ½ lemon
- 1 tablespoon walnuts, chopped

1. Put all ingredients in the blender.
2. Blend the smoothie until smooth.

per serving: 160 calories, 2.6g protein, 5.7g carbohydrates, 15.6g fat, 2.4g fiber, 0mg cholesterol, 32mg sodium, 329mg potassium.

Pistachio Smoothie

Prep time: 5 minutes | **Cook time:** 0 minutes | **Servings:** 4

- 2 oz pistachios
- 1 cup of coconut milk
- ½ cup oatmeal
- 1 tablespoon liquid honey

1. Mix coconut milk with oatmeal.
2. Meanwhile, blend pistachios with liquid honey and blend until smooth.
3. Add coconut milk mixture and blend the smoothie for 1 minute more.

per serving: 268 calories, 5.6g protein, 18.4g carbohydrates, 21.6g fat, 3.8g fiber, 0mg cholesterol, 85mg sodium, 344mg potassium.

Cayenne Pepper Smoothie

Prep time: 5 minutes | **Cook time:** 0 minutes | **Servings:** 4

- 1 teaspoon cayenne pepper
- 1 avocado, chopped
- ½ cup fresh spinach, chopped
- 1 cup of water
- 2 tablespoons coconut shred
- 1 cup of coconut milk

1. Blend cayenne pepper, avocado, spinach, water, coconut shred, and coconut milk until smooth.

per serving: 268 calories, 2.5g protein, 9g carbohydrates, 26.7g fat, 5.4g fiber, 0mg cholesterol, 18mg sodium, 432mg potassium.

Avocado and Beet Smoothie

Prep time: 5 minutes | **Cook time:** 0 minutes | **Servings:** 4

- 2 avocados, chopped
- 8 oz beets, peeled, chopped
- ½ cup of water
- 1 teaspoon ground paprika

1. Blend avocados with beets until smooth.
2. Add water and ground paprika.
3. Stir the smoothie.

per serving: 232 calories,2.9g protein, 14.6g carbohydrates, 19.8g fat, 8.1g fiber, 0mg cholesterol, 51mg sodium, 673mg potassium.

Tomato Smoothie

Prep time: 5 minutes | **Cook time:** 0 minutes | **Servings:** 4

- 2 cups tomatoes, chopped
- 1 avocado,
- chopped
- ½ teaspoon ground ginger

1. Blend tomatoes with avocado.
2. When the mixture is smooth, add ground ginger and carefully mix.
3. Pour the cooked smoothie in the glasses.

per serving: 120 calories,1.8g protein, 8g carbohydrates, 10g fat, 4.5g fiber, 0mg cholesterol, 7mg sodium, 460mg potassium.

Berries Tea

Prep time: 15 minutes | **Cook time:** 15 minutes | **Servings:** 4

- 2 tablespoons black tea
- 1 cup blueberries
- 5 cups of water

1. Bring the water to boil. Add blueberries. Simmer the mixture for 5 minutes.
2. Then blend the mixture, add black tea, and remove the drink from the heat.
3. Pour the drink in the cups.

per serving: 21 calories,0.3g protein, 5.3g carbohydrates, 0.1g fat, 0.9g fiber, 0mg cholesterol, 9mg sodium, 34mg potassium.

Apple Smoothie

Prep time: 5 minutes | **Cook time:** 0 minutes | **Servings:** 4

- 1 cup apples, chopped
- 1 cup apricots,
- chopped
- 1 cup of water

1. Blend apricots with apples and blend until smooth.
2. Add water and stir the smoothie.

per serving: 48 calories,0.7g protein, 12g carbohydrates, 0.4g fat, 2.1g fiber, 0mg cholesterol, 3mg sodium, 161mg potassium.

Tahini Smoothie

Prep time: 5 minutes | **Cook time:** 0 minutes | **Servings:** 4

- 2 tablespoons tahini paste
- 4 bananas, chopped
- 2 oranges, chopped
- ½ cup of water

1. Blend the ingredients in the blender.
2. When the mixture is smooth, pour it in the glasses.

per serving: 193 calories,3.4g protein, 39.4g carbohydrates, 4.5g fat, 6g fiber, 0mg cholesterol, 11mg sodium, 620mg potassium.

Lemonade

Prep time: 5 minutes | **Cook time:** 0 minutes | **Servings:** 4

- 4 cups of water
- 2 lemons, sliced
- 2 tablespoons mint
- Ice cubes

1. Mix water with lemon and mint.
2. Blend the mixture gently.
3. Pour it in the glasses and add ice cubes.

per serving: 10 calories,0.4g protein, 2.9g carbohydrates, 0.1g fat, 1g fiber, 0mg cholesterol, 9mg sodium, 55mg potassium.

Turmeric Smoothie

Prep time: 5 minutes | **Cook time:** 0 minutes | **Servings:** 2

- 1 tablespoon ground turmeric
- 1 cup of coconut milk
- 2 bananas, chopped
- 1 tablespoon fresh lemon juice

1. Put all ingredients in the blender.
2. Blend the smoothie well.

per serving: 395 calories,4.4g protein, 36g carbohydrates, 29.4g fat, 6.5g fiber, 0mg cholesterol, 22mg sodium, 833mg potassium.

Herbal Tea

Prep time: 15 minutes | **Cook time:** 10 minutes | **Servings:** 4

- 2 tablespoons herbal tea
- 1 orange, sliced
- 4 cups of water

1. Bring the water to boil.
2. Then remove it from the oven and add herbal tea and oranges.
3. Leave the tea for 15 minutes.

per serving: 22 calories,0.4g protein, 5.4g carbohydrates, 0.1g fat, 1.1g fiber, 0mg cholesterol, 7mg sodium, 86mg potassium.

Water with Herbs

Prep time: 25 minutes | **Cook time:** 0 minutes | **Servings:** 4

- 1 teaspoon rosemary
- 1 teaspoon mint
- 1 teaspoon
- chamomile
- 4 cups of water
- ½ lime

1. Pour water in the bottle.
2. Add all remaining ingredients and leave the drink for 15-20 minutes.

per serving: 4 calories,0.1g protein, 1.1g carbohydrates, 0.1g fat, 0.4g fiber, 0mg cholesterol, 8mg sodium, 16mg potassium.

Green Tea

Prep time: 15 minutes | **Cook time:** 10 minutes | **Servings:** 4

- 4 teaspoons green tea
- 1 tablespoon fresh mint
- 1 tablespoon lemon juice
- 4 cups of water

1. Bring the water to boil and add green tea.
2. Leave the tea for 10 minutes.
3. Then add mint and lemon juice.

per serving: 2 calories, 0.1g protein, 0.2g carbohydrates, 0g fat, 0.1g fiber, 0mg cholesterol, 8mg sodium, 14mg potassium.

Cinnamon Tea

Prep time: 15 minutes | **Cook time:** 15 minutes | **Servings:** 4

2 tablespoons green tea
- 4 cups of water
- 1 teaspoon ground
cinnamon

1. Bring water to boil.
2. Add green tea and stir the drink.
3. Then add ground cinnamon and pour it in the cups.

per serving: 1 calorie,0g protein, 0.5g carbohydrates, 0g fat, 0.3g fiber, 0mg cholesterol, 7mg sodium, 12mg potassium.

Green Tea with Lemon

Prep time: 5 minutes | **Cook time:** 15 minutes | **Servings:** 4

- 4 teaspoons green tea
- 4 lemon slices
- 4 cups of water

1. Bring the water to boil. Add green tea and remove the drink from the heat.
2. Then add lemon slices and pour the drink in the cups.

per serving: 2 calories,0.1g protein, 0.7g carbohydrates, 0g fat, 0.2g fiber, 0mg cholesterol, 7mg sodium, 27mg potassium.

Coconut Late

Prep time: 5 minutes | **Cook time:** 10 minutes | **Servings:** 4

- 4 teaspoons ground coffee
- 2 cups of coconut milk
- 1 cup of water
- 1 tablespoon shredded coconut

1. Bring the water to boil.
2. Add ground coffee and mix well.
3. Then pour the liquid in the glasses.
4. Add coconut milk and shredded coconut.

per serving: 280 calories,2.8g protein, 6.8g carbohydrates, 29g fat, 2.8g fiber, 0mg cholesterol, 20mg sodium, 323mg potassium.

Apple Tea

Prep time: 10 minutes | **Cook time:** 10 minutes | **Servings:** 4

- 4 lime slices
- 4 cups of water
- 1 cup apple, chopped

1. Pour water in the pan. Add lime and apple.
2. Simmer the apple tea for 10 minutes.

per serving: 30 calories,0.2g protein, 8.1g carbohydrates, 0.1g fat, 1.4g fiber, 0mg cholesterol, 8mg sodium, 65mg potassium.

Pears Chai

Prep time: 5 minutes | Cook time: 10 minutes | Servings: 4

- 1 tablespoon chai
- 4 pears, chopped
- 5 cups of water

1. 1. Mix water with chai and pears.
2. Bring the liquid to boil and simmer for 5-9 minutes.

per serving: 121 calories,0.8g protein, 31.8g carbohydrates, 0.3g fat, 6.5g fiber, 0mg cholesterol, 11mg sodium, 245mg potassium.

Cherry Drink

Prep time: 5 minutes | Cook time: 0 minutes | Servings: 4

- 5 cups of water
- 2 cups cherries
- 1 tablespoon liquid honey

1. Mix cherries with water and bring to boil.
2. Pour the drink in the glasses and add liquid honey.

per serving: 54 calories,0.8g protein, 13.8g carbohydrates, 0.3g fat, 1.3g fiber, 0mg cholesterol, 9mg sodium, 140mg potassium.

Mint Tea

Prep time: 10 minutes | Cook time: 10 minutes | Servings: 4

- 4 teaspoons black tea
- 4 teaspoons fresh
- mint
- 4 cups of water

1. Bring water to boil, add fresh mint.
2. Then remove the liquid from the heat, add black tea and stir well.
3. Pour the tea in the glasses.

per serving: 1 calorie, 0.1g protein, 0g carbohydrates, 0g fat, 0.1g fiber, 0mg cholesterol, 8mg sodium, 13mg potassium.

Mate Tea

Prep time: 15 minutes | Cook time: 10 minutes | Servings: 4

- 4 cups of water
- 2 tablespoons mate
- tea

1. Bring the water to boil.
2. Add mate tea and stir well.
3. Leave the tea for 10 minutes before serving.

per serving: 1 calorie,0g protein, 0.3g carbohydrates, 3g fat, 2g fiber, 0mg cholesterol, 7mg sodium, 2mg potassium.

Lime Drink

Prep time: 10 minutes | Cook time: 15 minutes | Servings: 4

- 3 cups of water
- 2 limes, chopped
- 1 tablespoon dried
- rosemary
- 2 tablespoons of liquid honey

1. Mix water with dried rosemary and bring to boil.
2. Remove the drink from the heat and add liquid honey and limes.

per serving: 45 calories,0.3g protein, 12.7g carbohydrates, 0.2g fat, 1.3g fiber, 0mg cholesterol, 7mg sodium, 49mg potassium.

Pumpkin Pie Tea

Prep time: 5 minutes | Cook time: 0 minutes | Servings: 4

- 4 teaspoons green tea
- 1 tablespoon
- pumpkin pie spices
- 4 cups of water

1. Bring water to boil and remove it from the heat.
2. Add green tea and leave the drink for 10 minutes.
3. Then add pumpkin pie spices and stir well.
4. Pour the drink in the cups.

per serving: 5 calories,0.1g protein, 1g carbohydrates, 0.2g fat, 0.2g fiber, 0mg cholesterol, 8mg sodium, 23mg potassium.

Berry Milkshake

Prep time: 5 minutes | **Cook time:** 0 minutes | **Servings:** 2

- 1 cup strawberries
- 1 cup blueberries
- 1 cup of coconut milk

1. Put all ingredients in the blender.
2. Blend the mixture until smooth.
3. Pour the cooked milkshake in the glasses.

per serving: 341 calories, 3.8g protein, 22.7g carbohydrates, 29.1g fat, 5.8g fiber, 0mg cholesterol, 19mg sodium, 482mg potassium.

Tropical Smoothie

Prep time: 5 minutes | **Cook time:** 0 minutes | **Servings:** 4

- 2 mangos, peeled, chopped
- 3 bananas, chopped
- 1 avocado, chopped
- ½ cup of coconut milk

1. Blend mangos with bananas and avocado.
2. Add coconut milk and pulse the smoothie for 5 seconds more.

per serving: 351 calories, 4g protein, 51.4g carbohydrates, 17.9g fat, 9g fiber, 0mg cholesterol, 10mg sodium, 922mg potassium.

Pineapple Smoothie

Prep time: 10 minutes | **Cook time:** 0 minutes | **Servings:** 4

- 1-pound pineapple, chopped
- 1 cup of coconut
- milk
- 1 avocado, chopped

1. Blend the pineapple with avocado until smooth.
2. Put the mixture in the glasses.
3. Add coconut milk and gently mix.

per serving: 297 calories, 2.9g protein, 22.5g carbohydrates, 24.2g fat, 6.3g fiber, 0mg cholesterol, 13mg sodium, 525mg potassium.

Apricot Smoothie

Prep time: 5 minutes | **Cook time:** 0 minutes | **Servings:** 4

- 2 cups apricots
- 3 tablespoons chia
- seeds
- 1 cup of water

1. Blend apricots with water until smooth.
2. Add chia seeds, gently mix, and pour the smoothie in the glasses.

per serving: 89 calories, 2.8g protein, 13g carbohydrates, 3.8g fat, 5.2g fiber, 0mg cholesterol, 4mg sodium, 245mg potassium.

Basil Tea

Prep time: 10 minutes | **Cook time:** 10 minutes | **Servings:** 4

- 4 lemon slices
- 1 cup fresh basil
- 4 cups of water

1. Bring water to boil.
2. Add basil and lemon slices.
3. Leave the tea for 10 minutes to rest.

per serving: 3 calories, 0.3g protein, 0.8g carbohydrates, 0.1g fat, 0.3g fiber, 0mg cholesterol, 7mg sodium, 30mg potassium.

Banana Smoothie

Prep time: 5 minutes | **Cook time:** 0 minutes | **Servings:** 4

- 1 avocado, chopped
- 4 bananas,
- chopped
- 1 cup of coconut milk

1. Put all ingredients in the blender and blend until smooth.
2. Pour the smoothie in the glasses.

per serving: 346 calories, 3.6g protein, 34.6g carbohydrates, 24.5g fat, 7.8g fiber, 0mg cholesterol, 13mg sodium, 824mg potassium.

Ginger and Cherry Smoothie

Prep time: 5 minutes | **Servings:** 4

- 1 oz fresh ginger, chopped
- ½ cup parsley,
- chopped
- 2 cups cherries
- ½ cup of water

1. Put all ingredients in the blender and blend until smooth.

per serving: 28 calories,0.9g protein, 5.6g carbohydrates, 0.5g fat, 1.2g fiber, 0mg cholesterol, 7mg sodium, 138mg potassium.

Kiwi Smoothie

Prep time: 5 minutes | **Servings:** 2

- 2 cups kiwi, peeled, chopped
- ½ cup of coconut milk

1. Put all ingredients in the blender and blend until smooth.
2. Pour the smoothie in the serving glasses.

per serving: 246 calories,3.4g protein, 29.3g carbohydrates, 15.2g fat, 6.6g fiber, 0mg cholesterol, 14mg sodium, 710mg potassium.

Masala Smoothie

Prep time: 10 minutes | **Servings:** 1

- ½ teaspoon garam masala
- ½ cup of coconut milk
- 2 bananas, chopped

1. Blend all ingredients in the blender.
2. Pour the smoothies in the serving glasses.

per serving: 486 calories, 29.4g protein, 60.6g carbohydrates, 29.4g fat, 8.8g fiber, 0mg cholesterol, 22mg sodium, 1160mg potassium.

Parsley Smoothie

Prep time: 10 minutes | **Servings:** 5

- 4 cups parsley, chopped
- 1 cup cilantro, chopped
- 1 cup of water
- 1 teaspoon ground black pepper
- 1 cup blueberries

1. Put all ingredients in the food processor and blend until smooth.
2. Pour the smoothies in the glasses.

per serving: 36 calories,1.8g protein, 7.6g carbohydrates, 0.5g fat, 2.5g fiber, 0mg cholesterol, 30mg sodium, 311mg potassium.

Almond Smoothie

Prep time: 5 minutes | **Cook time:** 0 minutes | **Servings:** 4

- ½ cup almonds, chopped
- 3 cups spinach, chopped
- 1 cup of coconut milk

1. Grind the almonds and blend them with spinach and coconut milk.
2. When the mixture is smooth, the drink is cooked.

per serving: 212 calories,4.5g protein, 6.7g carbohydrates, 20.3g fat, 3.3g fiber, 0mg cholesterol, 27mg sodium, 370mg potassium.

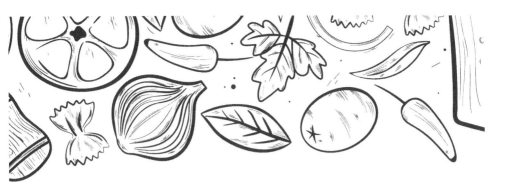

Desserts

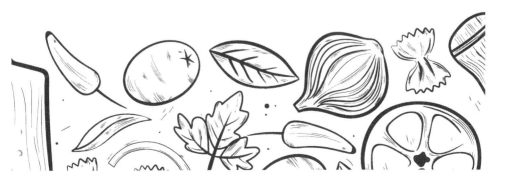

Baked Apples

Prep time: 10 minutes | **Cook time:** 15 minutes | **Servings:** 2

- 2 red apples
- 2 teaspoons honey

1. Cut the apples into halves and remove the seeds.
2. Then put the apple halves in the tray and bake at 400F for 15 minutes.
3. Sprinkle the apples with honey.

per serving: 137 calories, 0.6g protein, 36.6g carbohydrates, 0.4g fat, 5.4g fiber, 0mg cholesterol, 2mg sodium, 242mg potassium

Coconut Shake

Prep time: 10 minutes | **Cook time:** 0 minutes | **Servings:** 2

- 1 cup coconut cream
- 4 bananas, peeled, chopped
- 3 tablespoons coconut shred

1. Put all ingredients in the blender.
2. Blend the mixture until smooth.
3. Pour the dessert in the serving glasses.

per serving: 561 calories, 5.3g protein, 63.6g carbohydrates, 36.9g fat, 10.3g fiber, 0mg cholesterol, 24mg sodium, 1160mg potassium

Cinnamon Pears

Prep time: 15 minutes | **Cook time:** 10 minutes | **Servings:** 4

- 4 pears, halved
- 1 teaspoon ground cinnamon
- 1 teaspoon raw honey

1. Preheat the oven to 400F.
2. Then put the pears halves in the tray.
3. Sprinkle the fruits with ground cinnamon.
4. Bake the pears for 10 minutes.
5. Then top the cooked pears with raw honey.

per serving: 128 calories, 0.8g protein, 33.7g carbohydrates, 0.3g fat, 6.8g fiber, 0mg cholesterol, 3mg sodium, 246mg potassium

Strawberry Bowl

Prep time: 10 minutes | **Cook time:** 0 minutes | **Servings:** 4

- 3 cups strawberries, frozen
- 1 cup raspberries
- 1 teaspoon dried mint

1. Blend the strawberries until smooth.
2. Then mix the strawberry mixture with dried mint and raspberries.
3. Transfer the dessert in the bowls.

per serving: 51 calories, 1.1g protein, 12g carbohydrates, 0.5g fat, 4.2g fiber, 0mg cholesterol, 2mg sodium, 214mg potassium

Yogurt Pudding

Prep time: 25 minutes | **Cook time:** 0 minutes | **Servings:** 4

- 3 cups Plain yogurt
- 7 tablespoons chia seeds
- 2 oz raspberries

1. Mix plain yogurt with chia seeds and leave for 15 minutes.
2. Then transfer the pudding in the serving glasses and top with raspberries.

per serving: 241 calories, 14.1g protein, 23.6g carbohydrates, 8.9g fat, 8.2g fiber, 11mg cholesterol, 132mg sodium, 538mg potassium

Coconut Soufflé

Prep time: 20 minutes | **Cook time:** 0 minutes | **Servings:** 4

- 1 cup coconut cream
- 1 avocado, peeled, pitted, chopped
- 2 tablespoons coconut shred
- 1 teaspoon vanilla extract

1. Blend the avocado until smooth.
2. Then mix blended avocado with coconut cream.
3. Add coconut shred and vanilla extract. Stir the soufflé well.

per serving: 269 calories, 2.3g protein, 8.8g carbohydrates, 26.6g fat, 5.2g fiber, 0mg cholesterol, 13mg sodium, 403mg potassium

Cardamom Kiwis

Prep time: 10 minutes | **Cook time:** 10 minutes | **Servings:** 4

- 4 kiwis, halved
- 1 teaspoon ground cardamom
- 1 teaspoon almond butter

1. Sprinkle the kiwis with cardamom and put it in the tray.
2. Add almond butter and bake at 375F for 10 minutes.

per serving: 72 calories, 1.8g protein, 12.2g carbohydrates, 2.7g fat, 2.8g fiber, 0mg cholesterol, 3mg sodium, 273mg potassium

Peach Compote

Prep time: 10 minutes | **Cook time:** 20 minutes | **Servings:** 4

- 1 cup of water
- 3 cups peaches, pitted
- 1 teaspoon fresh mint
- 1 teaspoon honey

1. Bring the water to boil.
2. Add peaches and fresh mint.
3. Simmer the compote for 10 minutes.
4. Then remove the compote from the heat and cool to the room temperature.
5. Add honey and stir well.

per serving: 50 calories, 1.1g protein, 12g carbohydrates, 0.3g fat, 1.8g fiber, 0mg cholesterol, 2mg sodium, 217mg potassium

Quinoa Pudding

Prep time: 10 minutes | **Cook time:** 10 minutes | **Servings:** 4

- 3 cups of coconut milk
- 1 tablespoon almond flour
- 1 cup quinoa
- 2 bananas, chopped
- 1 tablespoon vanilla extract

1. Mix coconut milk with quinoa and almond flour.
2. Bring the mixture to boil and remove from the heat.
3. Add vanilla extract and bananas.
4. Stir the pudding well.

per serving: 643 calories, 11.1g protein, 51.5g carbohydrates, 46.5g fat, 8.7g fiber, 0mg cholesterol, 31mg sodium, 929mg potassium

Baked Peaches

Prep time: 10 minutes | **Cook time:** 10 minutes | **Servings:** 4

- 8 peaches, pitted, halved
- 1 tablespoon raw honey
- 1 teaspoon ground cinnamon

1. Put the peaches halves in the tray and sprinkle with ground cinnamon.
2. Bake the peaches for 10 minutes at 400F.

per serving: 135 calories, 2.8g protein, 32.8g carbohydrates, 0.8g fat, 4.9g fiber, 0mg cholesterol, 0mg sodium, 575mg potassium

Honey Cantaloupe

Prep time: 10 minutes | **Cook time:** 0 minutes | **Servings:** 4

- 3 cups cantaloupe
- 1 tablespoon liquid honey

1. Cut the cantaloupe into the cubes and put in the serving bowls.
2. Top the cantaloupe with liquid honey.

per serving: 56 calories, 1g protein, 13.9g carbohydrates, 0.2g fat, 1.1g fiber, 0mg cholesterol, 19mg sodium, 315mg potassium

Sweet Pumpkin

Prep time: 10 minutes | **Cook time:** 10 minutes | **Servings:** 4

- 2 tablespoons of liquid honey
- 4 cups pumpkin, chopped
- 1 teaspoon pumpkin pie spices

1. Mix pumpkin with pumpkin pie spices and liquid honey.
2. Leave the mixture for 10 minutes.
3. Then cook it on the medium heat for 10 minutes.
4. Cool the cooked pumpkin to the room temperature.

per serving: 117 calories, 2.8g protein, 28.8g carbohydrates, 0.7g fat, 7.2g fiber, 0mg cholesterol, 13mg sodium, 513mg potassium

Honey Strawberries

Prep time: 10 minutes | **Cook time:** 0 minutes | **Servings:** 4

- 2 cups strawberries
- 3 tablespoons raw honey
- 1 teaspoon lemon
- zest, grated
- 1 tablespoon lemon juice

1. Put the strawberries in the serving bowls.
2. Top the berries with raw honey, lemon zest, and lemon juice.

per serving: 72 calories, 0.6g protein, 18.7g carbohydrates, 0.3g fat, 1.5g fiber, 0mg cholesterol, 2mg sodium, 125mg potassium

Cinnamon Papaya

Prep time: 10 minutes | **Cook time:** 15 minutes | **Servings:** 4

- 2 cups papaya, roughly chopped
- 1 teaspoon ground
- cinnamon
- 1 tablespoon lemon juice

1. Put the papaya in the tray and sprinkle with ground cinnamon.
2. Bake the papaya for 15 minutes at 375F.
3. Sprinkle the cooked fruits with lemon juice.

per serving: 33 calories, 0.4g protein, 8.4g carbohydrates, 0.2g fat, 1.6g fiber, 0mg cholesterol, 7mg sodium, 139mg potassium

Rhubarb Bake

Prep time: 10 minutes | **Cook time:** 20 minutes | **Servings:** 6

- 3 cups rhubarb, chopped
- 1 teaspoon ground cinnamon
- 1 teaspoon lemon zest, grated
- 1 tablespoon almond butter

1. Line the baking tray with baking paper.
2. Then mix rhubarb with ground cinnamon, lemon zest, and almond butter.
3. Transfer the mixture in the baking tray, flatten it well, and bake at 365F for 20 minutes.

per serving: 30 calories, 1.2g protein, 3.7g carbohydrates, 1.6g fat, 1.6g fiber, 0mg cholesterol, 3mg sodium, 198mg potassium

Date Balls

Prep time: 10 minutes | **Cook time:** 0 minutes | **Servings:** 4

- 1 cup dates, chopped
- 1 oz pistachios,
- grinded
- 1 tablespoon lemon juice

1. Blend the dates with pistachios and lemon juice.
2. Make the balls from the date mixture.

per serving: 164 calories, 2.5g protein, 35.4g carbohydrates, 3.5g fat, 4.3g fiber, 0mg cholesterol, 39mg sodium, 370mg potassium

Strawberry Ice Cream

Prep time: 10 minutes | **Cook time:** 40 minutes | **Servings:** 4

- ½ cup coconut cream
- 3 cups
- strawberries, chopped

1. Blend the strawberries until smooth and mix with coconut cream.
2. Pour the mixture in the ice cream maker and cook according to the directions of the manufacturer.

per serving: 104 calories, 1.4g protein, 10g carbohydrates, 7.5g fat, 2.8g fiber, 0mg cholesterol, 6mg sodium, 244mg potassium

Avocado Ice Cream

Prep time: 10 minutes | **Cook time:** 40 minutes | **Servings:** 4

- 2 cups coconut cream
- 1 avocado, peeled,
- chopped
- 1 teaspoon ground ginger

1. Blend the avocado until smooth.
2. Then mix it with coconut cream and ground ginger.
3. Pour the mixture in the ice cream maker and cook according to the directions of the manufacturer.

per serving: 380 calories, 3.7g protein, 11.3g carbohydrates, 38.4g fat, 6.1g fiber, 0mg cholesterol, 21mg sodium, 556mg potassium

Baked Figs

Prep time: 10 minutes | **Cook time:** 20 minutes | **Servings:** 4

- 8 figs
- 1 oz pistachios, chopped
- 2 tablespoons of liquid honey

1. Make the crosswise cuts in the figs and fill them with pistachios.
2. Bake the figs at 375F for 20 minutes.
3. Sprinkle the cooked figs with liquid honey.

per serving: 164 calories, 2.7g protein, 34.8g carbohydrates, 3.7g fat, 4.5g fiber, 0mg cholesterol, 42mg sodium, 337mg potassium

Tropical Salad

Prep time: 10 minutes | **Cook time:** 0 minutes | **Servings:** 6

- 1 cup papaya, chopped
- 1 mango, chopped
- 2 kiwis, chopped
- 1 oz pistachios, chopped
- 2 tablespoons coconut cream

1. Put all ingredients in the serving bowl.
2. Gently shake the salad before serving.

per serving: 96 calories, 1.9g protein, 16.3g carbohydrates, 3.8g fat, 2.7g fiber, 0mg cholesterol, 29mg sodium, 279mg potassium

Orange Bowl

Prep time: 10 minutes | **Cook time:** 0 minutes | **Servings:** 4

- 3 nectarines, chopped
- 3 oranges, peeled, chopped
- 1 oz almonds, chopped
- 1 tablespoon raw honey

1. Mix nectarines with oranges and almonds.
2. Then put the ingredients in the serving bowls and top with raw honey.

per serving: 169 calories, 4g protein, 33.3g carbohydrates, 4.1g fat, 6g fiber, 0mg cholesterol, 0mg sodium, 519mg potassium

Ginger Mix

Prep time: 10 minutes | **Servings:** 6

- 3 tablespoons minced ginger
- 1 lemon, minced
- 1 tablespoon liquid honey

1. Put all ingredients in the can and carefully mix.
2. Close the lid and store the meal in the fridge for up to 7 days.

per serving: 23 calories, 0.4g protein, 5.7g carbohydrates, 0.2g fat, 0.6g fiber, 0mg cholesterol, 1mg sodium, 51mg potassium

Mango Sorbet

Prep time: 40 minutes | **Servings:** 4

- 2 mangoes, peeled and cubed
- ¼ cup of water

1. Blend the mangoes until smooth and mix with water.
2. Pour the mixture in the plastic vessel and freeze for 40 minutes.
3. Then blend the mixture until smooth and transfer in the serving bowls.

per serving: 101 calories, 1.4g protein, 25.2g carbohydrates, 0.6g fat, 2.7g fiber, 0mg cholesterol, 2mg sodium, 282mg potassium

Watermelon Juice

Prep time: 10 minutes | **Cook time:** 15 minutes | **Servings:** 4

- 3 cups watermelon
- 1 cup of orange juice

1. Blend the watermelon until smooth.
2. Then pour the orange juice in the ice mold and freeze until solid.
3. Pour the blended watermelon in the glasses.
4. Add orange juice cubes.

per serving: 62 calories, 1.1g protein, 15g carbohydrates, 0.3g fat, 0.6g fiber, 0mg cholesterol, 2mg sodium, 251mg potassium

Cherry Jam

Prep time: 10 minutes | **Cook time:** 10 minutes | **Servings:** 6

- 3 cups cherries, pitted, chopped
- 2 tablespoons honey

1. Mix the cherries with honey and saute the mixture for 10 minutes.
2. Transfer the jam in the glass cans and close the lids.

per serving: 71 calories, 0g protein, 17.8g carbohydrates, 0g fat, 0.5g fiber, 0mg cholesterol, 20mg sodium, 4mg potassium

Orange Ice

Prep time: 10 minutes | **Cook time:** 40 minutes | **Servings:** 4

- 4 cups orange juice
- 1 tablespoon liquid honey

1. Mix orange juice with liquid honey.
2. Then pour the mixture in the ice cube molds and freeze for 40 minutes.
3. Put the orange cubes in the food processor and blend until smooth.

per serving: 128 calories, 1.7g protein, 30.1g carbohydrates, 0.5g fat, 0.5g fiber, 0mg cholesterol, 2mg sodium, 499mg potassium

Oatmeal Pudding

Prep time: 10 minutes | **Cook time:** 30 minutes | **Servings:** 4

- 2 cups plain yogurt
- 1 cup oatmeal
- 1 teaspoon ground cinnamon
- 2 tablespoons of liquid honey

1. Mix plain yogurt with oatmeal and ground cinnamon.
2. Leave the mixture for 30 minutes.
3. Then put the pudding in the serving glasses and top with liquid honey.

per serving: 198 calories, 9.7g protein, 31.6g carbohydrates, 2.8g fat, 2.4g fiber, 7mg cholesterol, 87mg sodium, 369mg potassium

Peach Pudding

Prep time: 10 minutes | **Cook time:** 10 minutes | **Servings:** 4

- 2 cups peaches, pitted, chopped
- 1 cup coconut cream
- 2 tablespoons almond flour
- 1 teaspoon vanilla extract

1. Bring the coconut cream to boil and add the almond flour.
2. Simmer the liquid for 5 minutes.
3. Then blend the peaches until smooth and add in the coconut cream mixture.
4. Stir well and transfer the pudding in the serving bowls.

per serving: 192 calories, 2.8g protein, 11.2g carbohydrates, 16.2g fat, 2.9g fiber, 0mg cholesterol, 10mg sodium, 302mg potassium

Chia and Banana Pudding

Prep time: 10 minutes | **Cook time:** 0 minutes | **Servings:** 3

- 1 cup coconut cream
- 4 tablespoons chia seeds
- 2 bananas, chopped

1. Blend the bananas until smooth and mix them with coconut cream and chia seeds.
2. Pour the pudding into the serving bowls.

per serving: 346 calories, 5.8g protein, 30.4g carbohydrates, 25.1g fat, 10.3g fiber, 0mg cholesterol, 16mg sodium, 569mg potassium

Strawberry Compote

Prep time: 10 minutes | **Cook time:** 20 minutes | **Servings:** 6

- 3 cups strawberries chopped
- 1 cup apricots,
- 2 cups of water

1. Bring the water to boil and add strawberries.
2. Then add apricots and simmer the meal for 10 minutes.
3. Cool the compote and pour it into glasses.

per serving: 35 calories, 0.8g protein, 8.4g carbohydrates, 0.4g fat, 1.9g fiber, 0mg cholesterol, 3mg sodium, 178mg potassium

Blackberry Pudding

Prep time: 10 minutes | **Cook time:** 0 minutes | **Servings:** 6

- 3 cups blackberries
- 1 cup coconut cream
- 1 tablespoon chia seeds

1. Blend the blackberries until smooth and mix them with chia seeds and coconut cream.
2. Pour the pudding in the serving glasses.

per serving: 134 calories, 2.3g protein, 10.1g carbohydrates, 10.6g fat, 5.5g fiber, 0mg cholesterol, 7mg sodium, 231mg potassium

Baked Apricot Halves

Prep time: 10 minutes | **Cook time:** 15 minutes | **Servings:** 4

Ingredients:8 apricots, halved
- 1 teaspoon ground cinnamon
- 1 oz almonds, chopped

1. Put the apricot halves in the tray in one layer.
2. Top the fruits with ground cinnamon and almonds.
3. Bake the dessert for 15 minutes at 365F.

per serving: 76 calories, 2.4g protein, 9.7g carbohydrates, 4g fat, 2.6g fiber, 0mg cholesterol, 1mg sodium, 236mg potassium

Chia Bars

Prep time: 20 minutes | **Cook time:** 0 minutes | **Servings:** 4

- 3 oz chia seeds
- 6 dates, chopped
- 3 oz walnuts, chopped
- 1 teaspoon lemon zest, grated
- 1 teaspoon honey

Method:

1. In the mixing bowl, mix chia seeds with dates, walnuts, lemon zest, and honey.
2. Mix the mixture until smooth.
3. Then roll it up in the shape of the square and cut into bars.

per serving: 275 calories, 9g protein, 21.9g carbohydrates, 19.1g fat, 9.8g fiber, 0mg cholesterol, 4mg sodium, 282mg potassium

Chocolate Mousse

Prep time: 10 minutes | **Cook time:** 0 minutes | **Servings:** 4

- 1 avocado, pitted, peeled, chopped
- 1 tablespoon cocoa powder
- ¼ cup coconut cream

1. Blend the avocado with cocoa powder.
2. When the mixture is smooth, add coconut cream.
3. Pulse the mousse for 2 minutes more.

per serving: 140 calories, 1.5g protein, 5.9g carbohydrates, 13.6g fat, 4.1g fiber, 0mg cholesterol, 6mg sodium, 317mg potassium

Carrot Soufflé

Prep time: 10 minutes | **Cook time:** 25 minutes | **Servings:** 4

- 2 cups carrot, grated
- 4 eggs, beaten
- ½ cup coconut cream
- 1 tablespoon liquid honey

1. Mix eggs with carrot, coconut cream, and liquid honey.
2. Transfer the mixture in the baking cups and bake at 365F for 25 minutes.

per serving: 170 calories, 6.7g protein, 11.7g carbohydrates, 11.5g fat, 2g fiber, 164mg cholesterol, 104mg sodium, 316mg potassium

Baked Bananas

Prep time: 10 minutes | **Cook time:** 15 minutes | **Servings:** 6

- 6 bananas, halved
- 1 teaspoon ground cinnamon
- 1 teaspoon vanilla extract
- 1 tablespoon almond butter

1. Rub the banana halves with ground cinnamon, vanilla extract, and almond butter.
2. Put the bananas in the tray and bake at 365F for 15 minutes.

per serving: 124 calories, 1.9g protein, 27.9g carbohydrates, 1.9g fat, 3.5g fiber, 0mg cholesterol, 1mg sodium, 445mg potassium

Pomegranate Pudding

Prep time: 10 minutes | **Cook time:** 20 minutes | **Servings:** 4

- 1 cup oatmeal
- 2 cups of coconut milk
- 3 almond butter
- ½ cup pomegranate seeds

Bring the coconut milk to boil.

1. Add oatmeal and almond butter.
2. Simmer the mixture for 5 minutes.
3. Then remove it from the heat, add pomegranate seeds and stir well.
4. Transfer the pudding in the serving bowls.

per serving: 440 calories, 8.1g protein, 25.7g carbohydrates, 36.7g fat, 6g fiber, 0mg cholesterol, 20mg sodium, 480mg potassium

Mango Pudding

Prep time: 10 minutes | **Cook time:** 0 minutes | **Servings:** 2

- 1 mango, peeled, blended
- 1 cup plain yogurt
- 3 oz chia seeds
- 1 teaspoon fresh mint

1. Mix plain yogurt with chia seeds and put in the serving glasses.
2. Top the yogurt with fresh mint and blended mango.

per serving: 395 calories, 15.4g protein, 51.8g carbohydrates, 15.2g fat, 17.4g fiber, 7mg cholesterol, 95mg sodium, 746mg potassium

Matcha Pudding

Prep time: 10 minutes | **Cook time:** 10 minutes | **Servings:** 4

- 1 teaspoon matcha powder
- 1 cup coconut cream
- 2 oz chia seeds
- 1 tablespoon liquid honey

1. Mix matcha powder with coconut cream and bring to boil.
2. Then cool the mixture, add chia seeds and liquid honey.
3. Stir the pudding well.

per serving: 224 calories, 4g protein, 13.6g carbohydrates, 18.7g fat, 6.5g fiber, 0mg cholesterol, 11mg sodium, 225mg potassium

Pineapple Sorbet

Prep time: 50 minutes | **Cook time:** 0 minutes | **Servings:** 4

- 2 tablespoons of liquid honey
- 1 teaspoon fresh
- mint
- 2 cups pineapple, chopped

1. Blend the pineapple until smooth.
2. Add liquid honey and mint. Stir the mixture.
3. • Put the mixture in the silicone molds and freeze for 40 minutes.
4. Then remove the mixture from the molds, transfer in the food processor and blend until smooth.
5. Put the dessert in the serving bowls.

per serving: 73 calories, 0.5g protein, 19.5g carbohydrates, 0.1g fat, 1.2g fiber, 0mg cholesterol, 2mg sodium, 98mg potassium

Pumpkin Balls

Prep time: 10 minutes | **Cook time:** 0 minutes | **Servings:** 4

- 4 oz pumpkin seeds, crushed
- 1 oz chia seeds
- 5 dates, chopped
- 1 teaspoon honey

1. Put all ingredients in the mixing bowl and mix until smooth.
2. Make the small balls from the mixture and store them in the fridge for up to 4 days.

per serving: 222 calories, 8.4g protein, 17.3g carbohydrates, 15.2g fat, 4.4g fiber, 0mg cholesterol, 7mg sodium, 327mg potassium

Stuffed Dates

Prep time: 10 minutes | **Cook time:** 0 minutes | **Servings:** 4

- 8 dates, pitted
- 8 almonds

1. Fill the dates with almonds.
2. Store the dates up to 4 days in the fridge.

per serving: 61 calories, 0.9g protein, 13g carbohydrates, 1.3g fat, 1.6g fiber, 0mg cholesterol, 0mg sodium, 126mg potassium

Cinnamon Brown Rice Pudding

Prep time: 10 minutes | **Cook time:** 20 minutes | **Servings:** 5

- 3 cups of coconut milk
- 1 cup of brown rice
- 1 tablespoon liquid honey
- 1 teaspoon cinnamon powder

1. Mix coconut milk with brown rice and ground cinnamon.
2. Simmer the mixture for 20 minutes on low heat.
3. Then remove the pudding from the heat, cool little, add liquid honey, and stir the pudding well.

per serving: 482 calories, 6.2g protein, 40.4g carbohydrates, 35.4g fat, 4.5g fiber, 0mg cholesterol, 23mg sodium, 483mg potassium

Melon Sorbet

Prep time: 45 minutes | **Cook time:** 0 minutes | **Servings:** 4

- 4 cups melon, chopped
- ¼ cup coconut cream

1. Blend the melon until smooth.
2. Mix the melon with coconut cream and pour the mixture in the plastic vessel.
3. Freeze the sorbet for 40 minutes.
4. Then blend the sorbet gently and put in the serving plates.

per serving: 88 calories, 1.7g protein, 13.6g carbohydrates, 3.9g fat, 1.7g fiber, 0mg cholesterol, 27mg sodium, 456mg potassium

Blueberries Sorbet

Prep time: 50 minutes | **Cook time:** 0 minutes | **Servings:** 6

- 4 cups blueberries
- ¼ cup apple juice
- 1 teaspoon honey

1. Blend the blueberries until smooth and mix the mixture with apple juice and honey.
2. Freeze the mixture until solid and then blend with the help of the food processor.

per serving: 64 calories, 0.7g protein, 16.1g carbohydrates, 0.3g fat, 2.4g fiber, 0mg cholesterol, 1mg sodium, 85mg potassium

Apple Jam

Prep time: 10 minutes | **Cook time:** 25 minutes | **Servings:** 4

- 4 apples, peeled, chopped
- 1 teaspoon ground cinnamon
- 1 tablespoon lemon juice

1. Mix the apples with lemon juice and ground cinnamon.
2. Put the mixture in the baking pan and cook for 25 minutes at 360F. Stir the mixture from time to time to avoid burning.
3. Then blend the cooked jam and transfer it in the cans.

per serving: 118 calories, 0.7g protein, 0g carbohydrates, 0.4g fat, 5.7g fiber, 0mg cholesterol, 3mg sodium, 246mg potassium

Grilled Pineapple

Prep time: 10 minutes | **Cook time:** 5 minutes | **Servings:** 6

- 3 cups pineapple, roughly chopped
- ½ teaspoon ground ginger
- 1 tablespoon coconut cream

1. Preheat the grill to 400F.
2. Then sprinkle the pineapple with ground ginger and put in the grill.
3. Cook it for 2 minutes per side.
4. Top the cooked pineapple with coconut cream.

per serving: 47 calories, 0.5g protein, 11.1g carbohydrates, 0.7g fat, 1.2g fiber, 0mg cholesterol, 1mg sodium, 99mg potassium

Sweet Grape Salad

Prep time: 10 minutes | **Cook time:** 0 minutes | **Servings:** 4

- 2 cups green grapes
- 1 cup strawberries, chopped
- 1 tablespoon coconut shred
- 1 teaspoon ground cinnamon
- 2 tablespoons coconut cream

1. In the mixing bowl, mix green grapes, strawberries, coconut shred, and ground cinnamon.

2. Top the salad with coconut cream.

per serving: 74 calories, 0.7g protein, 12.1g carbohydrates, 3.3g fat, 1.9g fiber, 0mg cholesterol, 3mg sodium, 165mg potassium

Mango Bowl

Prep time: 10 minutes | **Cook time:** 0 minutes | **Servings:** 4

- 2 mangos, pitted, peeled, chopped
- 2 kiwis, peeled, chopped
- 1 cup watermelon, chopped

1. Put all ingredients in the bowl.
2. Gently shake the ingredients.

per serving: 135 calories, 2g protein, 33.6g carbohydrates, 0.9g fat, 4g fiber, 0mg cholesterol, 3mg sodium, 443mg potassium

Watermelon Sorbet

Prep time: 35 minutes | **Cook time:** 0 minutes | **Servings:** 6

- 4 cups watermelon
- 1 teaspoon fresh mint

1. Blend the watermelon until smooth.
2. Then put in the freezer and freeze for 30 minutes.
3. Then blend the sorbet well and mix with mint.

per serving: 31 calories, 0.6g protein, 7.6g carbohydrates, 0.1g fat, 0.4g fiber, 0mg cholesterol, 1mg sodium, 114mg potassium

Measurement Conversion Charts

Measurement

Cup	Ounces	Milliliters	Tablespoons
8 cups	64 oz	1895	128
6 cups	48 oz	1420	96
5 cups	40 oz	1180	80
4 cups	32 oz	960	64
2 cups	16 oz	480	32
1 cups	8 oz	240	16
3/4 cups	6 oz	177	12
2/3 cups	5 oz	158	11
1/2 cups	4 oz	118	8
3/8 cups	3 oz	90	6
1/3 cups	2.5 oz	79	5.5
1/4 cups	2 oz	59	4
1/8 cups	1 oz	30	3
1/16 cups	1/2 oz	15	1

Weight

Imperial	Metric
1/2 oz	15 g
1 oz	29 g
2 oz	57 g
3 oz	85 g
4 oz	113 g
5 oz	141 g
6 oz	170 g
8 oz	227 g
10 oz	283 g
12 oz	340 g
13 oz	369 g
14 oz	397 g
15 oz	425 g
1 lb	453 g

Temperature

Fahrenheit	Celsius
100 °F	37 °C
150 °F	65 °C
200 °F	93 °C
250 °F	121 °C
300 °F	150 °C
325 °F	160 °C
350 °F	180 °C
375 °F	190 °C
400 °F	200 °C
425 °F	220 °C
450 °F	230 °C
500 °F	260 °C
525 °F	274 °C
550 °F	288 °C

Recipe Index

Barley Soup, 47

beans
Sprouts Salad, 22
Cayenne Pepper Green Beans, 30
Rosemary Black Beans, 31
Oregano Green Beans, 32
Beans Mash, 34
Bean Soup, 46
Okra Salad, 63
Chicken and Beans, 69
Chicken with Green Beans, 70
Mint Green Beans, 92
Garlic Green Beans, 93
Poached Green Beans, 95
Bean Spread, 96

beet
Horseradish Sauce, 107
Beet Noodles Salad, 23
Beet Soup, 47
Chicken and Beets, 71
Mint and Beet Smoothie, 113
Avocado and Beet Smoothie, 116

bell pepper
Pepper Eggs, 19
Chicken with Peppers, 69
Stuffed Peppers with Cod, 87

blackberries
Crab Salad, 57
Blackberries Smoothie, 114
Blackberry Pudding, 128

blueberries
Blueberry Bowl, 20
Blueberry Porridge, 23
Berries BBQ Sauce, 104
Cinnamon and Blueberries Smoothie, 114
Berries Tea, 116
Berry Milkshake, 119
Parsley Smoothie, 120
Blueberries Sorbet, 130

bok choy
Lemon Bok Choy, 94

broccoli
Baked Broccoli, 29
Cheesy Broccoli, 32
Glazed Broccoli, 32
Broccoli Puree, 37
Tomato Soup, 41
Broccoli Soup, 41
Coconut Soup, 42
Chard Soup, 44
Barley Soup, 47
Broccoli Steaks, 94

brussel sprouts
Turmeric Salad, 59
Vegetable Roast, 91
Cilantro Brussels Sprouts, 30
Lime Brussels Sprouts, 31

bulgur
Bulgur Salad, 62

butter
Green Peas Paste, 95
Peanut Dressing, 104
Peanut Dressing, 110
Baked Bananas, 128

butternut squash
Baked Butternut Squash, 97

c

cabbage
Cabbage Salad, 20
Cabbage Bowl, 31
Easy Cabbage Slaw, 34
Cabbage Steaks, 36
Red Soup, 44
Slaw, 56
Mint Salad, 56
Napa Cabbage Salad, 60
Chicken and Cabbage Bowl, 74

calamari
Tomato Calamari, 85

cantaloupe
Cantaloupe Salad, 58
Honey Cantaloupe, 124

carambola
Apple Salad, 56

carrot
Winter Salad, 19
Shredded Carrot Bowl, 22
Lemon Carrots, 29
Rosemary Carrots, 29
Easy Cabbage Slaw, 34
Broccoli Soup, 41
Spinach Soup, 43
Green Peas Soup, 43
Cumin Soup, 45
Slaw, 56
Chicken Alfredo, 75
Cod with Carrot, 83
Salmon and Carrot Balls, 87
Scallop Stew, 87
Vegetable Roast, 91
Baked Leek, 94
Carrot Soufflé, 128
Spiralized Carrot, 34
Ginger Cauliflower Soup, 42
Meatball Soup, 45
Carrot Salad, 59
Zucchini Salad, 61
Noodle Salad, 62
Thyme Carrots, 91
Carrot Noodles, 93

cashew
Cashew Sauce, 106

cauliflower
Cauliflower Puree, 30
Ginger Cauliflower Soup, 42
Cauliflower Cream Soup, 46
Beet Soup, 47
Parsnip Cream Soup, 49
Sorrel Soup, 49
Cauliflower Steaks, 91
Cauliflower Balls, 97

celery
Winter Salad, 19
Baked Celery Root, 36
Celery Cream Soup, 48
Celery Stalk Salad, 60
Baked Celery Root, 99

chamomile
Water with Herbs, 117